HOW
TO FEEL
BETTER

HOW TO FEEL BETTER

Boost Your Immune System and Reduce Inflammation for Lifelong Health and Vitality

NICK HALL, PhD

MEDIA

Published 2019 by Gildan Media LLC
aka G&D Media
www.GandDmedia.com

FIRST EDITION 2019

Front Cover design by David Rheinhardt of Pyrographx

Interior design by Meghan Day Healey of Story Horse, LLC

Library of Congress Cataloging-in-Publication Data is available upon
request

ISBN: 978-1-7225-0016-0

10   9   8   7   6   5   4   3   2   1

Contents

Introduction

Every day we are exposed to bacteria and viruses. We put things into our bodies on the backs of forks, toothbrushes. We inhale the air that is being expelled by people who cough and sneeze around us. Some of the viruses we are exposed to have the potential of triggering illness; many are perfectly harmless. The purpose of this book is to describe ways of staying well and avoiding symptoms, despite the fact that every day we are exposed to pathogens which are everywhere.

When you wipe the corner of your eye you are transferring the virus you've come into contact with to the biological equivalent of the Club Med. The temperature, the humidity in the corner of your eye and your nasal passages are absolutely ideal. It doesn't take long for the virus to wend its way into the genetic machinery of your healthy cells, soon to transform those cells into miniature factories which will later produce copious amounts of that same virus, so that three to five days later you'll have a scratchy throat, a runny nose, the classic manifestations of a cold.

However, even when we are exposed to potentially dangerous microbes we rarely succumb to those symptoms. Many people are not even aware that they came close to developing an illness and that is because their immune system was robust enough to protect them from those symptoms. They stayed in what is referred to as the pre- or subclinical phase.

There are things that happen to us that unfortunately prevent the immune system from doing its job. Chronic emotional upheaval, otherwise known as stress, will produce chemicals in your body that will drive down your immune system, leaving you susceptible to the symptoms associated with those microbes we happen to encounter. Or sometimes you might be overwhelmed with a very large amount of a particularly virulent microbe overwhelming even a robust immune system.

The focus of this book is the immune system and how to prevent the symptoms of inflammation from overwhelming us. We will look at the ways you can maintain an optimal state of immunity in order to prevent symptoms from occurring, and for those times when you happen to experience symptoms, how to use nutrition and very simple behavioral techniques to feel better much more quickly.

The Basics—
Prepare Your Body

I t is pointless to take steps to fine-tune the immune system unless you first prepare your body in a general way. What is good for the brain, is good for the heart, is good for the endocrine system, and each of these impacts the immune system. Therefore, you have to take care of the basics before trying to fine-tune your white cells in order to optimize them. Of all the things we can do to maintain an optimal state of overall good health, the most important is to pay attention to what you eat.

A healthful diet is absolutely essential. Although getting adequate sleep and movement through exercise are absolutely paramount as well, I'd like to begin by talking about the things that can be done with a knife and fork in order to maintain a good foundation of good health.

First of all a healthful diet has to be adequate and by that I mean it must provide the energy substrates that are required. Foods that are rich in carbohydrates as well as fat are the primary sources of energy for the body. At the same time our diet must meet the cell's requirements for what we call micronutrients, including vitamins, minerals and fiber. Adequate levels of all of these are critically important, and if a person does not consume enough then all of the systems that help maintain optimal health are going to fail.

A healthful diet is also moderate. Moderation refers to consuming the different sources of micro and macronutrients in just the right amount. You don't want too much nor do you want too little. In both biology and medicine, more is not better. What we need is to be in that optimal midrange. If a person consumes too much carbohydrate, too much fat, too much protein, there will be severe consequences, just as there will be if a person does not consume enough of these. A healthful diet is going to be balanced and that means it is going to provide the right proportions of all of the different ingredients that you need.

There are lots of different things that are needed by the immune system especially. You need adequate amounts of vitamin C and vitamin A. You also need adequate protein since antibodies, which are produced by our lymphocytes, are made of protein. For enzymatic reactions, the chemical processes that enable the entire system to function, we require iron, zinc, copper, and many other minerals.

And finally, a healthful diet is going to be varied, which means eating many different types of foods. A very good way of doing this is to make sure there's a lot of color on your plate. The color reflects the phytochem-icals that are present in vegetables and fruits. The more variety you have, the more of these different colors in your meals, the more of these ingredients you are get-ting.

Some of these phytochemicals have been found to be protective against cancer. They benefit you in staving off heart disease and they work in a number of ways to maintain an optimal state of immunity. When one thinks about nutrition and food then the word calories comes to mind. You need a certain number of calories in order to provide the energy that cells require in order to perform their various functions.

Problems arise when too much calorie or energy-laden food is consumed which does not provide ade-quate amounts of nutrients and micronutrients. It's very important to make sure that you consume fewer empty calories, those calories from foods and beverages that are missing these critical ingredients for optimal cell functioning. As you take steps to mobilize your immune system by ingesting the right types of foods, there are certain things that you do not want to overdue.

For example, excessive consumption of sodium which is found in the salt we put on our foods. It's also an ingre-dient in many of the processed foods that we purchase over the counter. This can lead to high blood pressure in some people, but not all. It can also cause some people to lose calcium from their bones rendering them suscep-tible to osteoporosis, as well as other problems with the skeletal system.

Fat is essential, you need a certain amount of fat to cushion organs. You need fat to help regulate the balance of steroids. This is particularly important in women. The fat which accumulates in the hip region helps to regulate the balance of estrogen and progesterone. Female athletes who do not consume enough fat and do not have sufficient fat in this region often will have abnormal reproductive cycles and may even stop menstruating.

However, too much fat, especially in the form of saturated fats, can leave one susceptible to coronary arterial disease. As I said earlier, we don't ever want too much of any single ingredient. It's also important to limit the consumption of refined sugars. People who consume too much sugar in sweetened soft drinks, fruit drinks, baked goods such as cookies and cakes are quite likely to experience overweight and obesity and are more likely to have dental caries and other problems indicative of tooth decay.

Alcohol does provide energy, though it contains kilocalories, not nutrients. We tend to refer to alcohol as containing empty calories. The temptation to consume things that we don't really need is one of the more important problems we face in maintaining an optimal diet.

There is a difference between appetite and hunger. Appetite is a psychological term. It's the desire to eat a certain food, whereas hunger is driven by a physiological need. For example you experience hunger pains when you haven't eaten for some time. Hunger is very difficult to exert control over; your body is demanding that you ingest a certain number of calories.

However, it is possible to exert control over appetite. When you've had breakfast and then walk by your favorite bakery with that succulent cake sitting in the window, although you don't really need those calories your appetite is telling you, "I really want to consume that." It's in this arena of appetite where you can take conscious steps to maintain optimal body weight, as well as to provide the right balance of ingredients for your physiological systems to work optimally.

For example there are some foods that are very low in nutrients. A person who eats a breakfast of puffed rice cereal with a cup of whole milk and a slice of white toast with a tablespoon of butter is getting relatively low nutrients. They're getting plenty of energy, that white refined bread in the toast is very high on the glycemic index. Blood sugar goes up very quickly, since carbohydrate is made of basically glucose.

An alternative breakfast which provides high nutrient density would be cooked oatmeal, instead of the puffed rice cereal, a half cup of skim milk instead of the cup of whole milk and a slice of whole wheat toast instead of the white toast.

One can still enjoy a mid-day snack, but instead of a soft drink with a piece of cheese, try a peeled orange with nonfat yogurt. A hamburger can be replaced with a turkey sandwich and a chocolate chip cookie with half a whole wheat bagel. A green salad comprised of diced tomatoes, green onions, bacon bits, ranch salad dressing could be replaced with fresh spinach leaves, green peppers, kidney beans, and fat-free Italian salad dressing.

These are just some very simple examples with common foods that a lot of people eat. These substitutions will provide the same number of calories along with the nutrients required to maintain optimal health. The general idea is to increase your intake of fruits and vegetables, and try to eat a variety of different colored vegetables along with legumes, such as beans and peas. Make sure that at least half of the grain foods that you eat are made from whole grains, including breads, cereals and pasta.

Whenever possible choose milk and milk products that are fat-free or low-fat. And when choosing proteins you'll be a lot better off choosing those lower in solid fat and calories, for example, lean cuts of beef or skinless poultry. It's not a bad idea to include more fish and shellfish in your diet as a substitute for some of the traditional red meat and poultry choices that are commonly made in America. I would also recommend choosing eggs, beans, peas, soy products, and unsalted nuts and seeds.

Here are some tips that will enable you to still enjoy food. We need a certain amount of pleasure in life and eating good tasty food is one important way of doing that. We can focus on the choices you can make. For example, I like to avoid those all-you-can-eat, belly-up-to-the-buffet restaurants. There's just too much temptation to consume way too much.

I avoid those appetizers that are breaded and especially those that are fried or, as is very popular today, filled with cheese or meat. In fact you might consider just skipping the appetizer completely and choosing a salad or something else. I like to order broth-based soups instead of cream-based and instead of a beef burger, order a chicken or veggie burger or a fish sandwich.

Instead of eating the entire meal yourself ask for a single entree with two plates and split it with a friend. Check out the children's menu, which is often a smaller portion. Another option is to order a healthful appetizer instead of the larger meal, or perhaps a combination of appetizers.

Order a salad that comes with low fat or nonfat dressing served on the side. What you really want is the flavor in the dressing, so you don't need to place it over the entire salad. Simply dipping your fork into the dressing before stabbing that piece of lettuce or carrot will provide you with just the right amount of flavor from the dressing, without consuming all those extra calories. You'll be absolutely amazed at how much you enjoyed that salad, yet at the end the little bowl of dressing on the side is still nearly full.

You don't have to eat everything on your plates. I know many people grew up as members of the clean-plate club. They were told that if they didn't consume every morsel of food on their plate then some poor child in Africa would starve to death. That absolutely is not true. When you feel full, when you reach the point where you don't need any more food that is when you take the rest home for another meal.

Dessert doesn't have to be death by chocolate. Dessert could be a piece of fruit. It might be an after-dinner beverage, such as a cup of tea. It's always nice to have something that finishes off a meal and even something sweet, but it doesn't have to be a fatty dessert. It can be something that is healthful as well. These are just some of the things that you can do to continue to enjoy eating while improving your intake of healthy nutrients.

Another important aspect to fueling your immunity is to avoid exposure to microbes. As I noted before, we put things into our mouths on forks, toothbrushes and our hands, and should realize that the oral cavity, the mouth, is the primary portal for most microbes entering the body. It is especially important to make sure that the foods you eat are as free as possible of microbial organisms. That means washing your hands, any food contact surface, as well as the fruits and vegetables you are going to consume.

A lot of people feel that if they are eating organic they don't have to worry about washing off the pesticides. Farmers who grow organic foods use natural fertilizer which could mean fecal matter from animals is being used as the fertilizer. You need to wash those vegetables very carefully and completely to make sure that you don't end up with E. coli or salmonella, or other nasty microbes that might cause illness.

Make sure that you keep separated raw and cooked foods. While shopping, you might separate foods that will need to be refrigerated and those that don't. You certainly want to avoid contact between a raw, uncooked food and something you might be consuming as is, such as a head of lettuce. Make sure that foods are cooked to a safe temperature and be sure to chill perishable foods as promptly as possible.

If you don't want to keep track of all of this, just think Mediterranean diet. Without question the most healthful diet on the planet, Mediterranean diets have been found to be associated with decreased depression, lower heart disease, as well as lower instances of inflammation, such as These are typically consumed in areas who boarder the Mediterranean Sea, including Portugal, Spain, southern Italy, Israel, Turkey and Lebanon. It's the opposite of the average American diet.

For example, red meat is not consumed on a daily basis, or even on a weekly basis. Red meat is eaten only once a month. Eggs, fish, and poultry are only eaten a few days each week, and beans, nuts and seeds are abundant throughout. Making the diet low in saturated fats and refined sugars is the real objective here.

When preparing these foods, mainly olive oil is used, making the diet rich in monounsaturated fats. Foods eaten daily are those that provide you with energy. Carbohydrates, including bread, pasta, couscous, fruits, beans, and other legumes are an integral part of the Mediterranean diet, as are nuts, vegetables, cheese, and yogurt. These choices make this diet very high in all of the vitamins and minerals that you need as well as providing fiber, phytochemicals, as well as probiotics, small amounts of the good bacteria that we need to help with digestion and have been found to help ward off inflammation, as well as prebiotics, the things that the bacteria need in order to maintain healthful populations.

I might add that wine is included in moderation as part of the Mediterranean diet, note *in moderation*. Resveratrol, an ingredient in very dark red wine, has been found to have anticancer properties. The flavonoids found in wine are antioxidants. There are health benefits, but in moderation.

Realize that alcohol is a toxin and in large amounts it can interfere with the enzymatic processes taking place in the liver, and can damage parts of the brain that we need to consolidate information into memory. That part of the brain is the hippocampus.

Alcohol in excess can interfere with relationships, productivity, and can certainly cause other obstacles to a healthy lifestyle.

But our rally is everything in moderation. Consuming a small amount of wine is a critical part of the Mediterranean diet and some health benefits are obtained. This type of dietary regimen will provide you with the foundation for optimal health.

Meet Your Immune System

f you are going to stay well and feel better, you really have to pay attention to your immune system. That is the system that protects us from those constant ubiquitous microbes that we live with from the moment we are born until the day we die. One of the things that will impair the immune system, perhaps more than anything else, is emotional upheaval.

Realize there are some people who are not fazed by stress; they seem to thrive on it. They seek out occupations that result in their being surrounded by stressful events. These include, for example, law enforcement, fire fighters, and people who volunteer for the military. There are certain characteristics that distinguish a person who is able to maintain a state of optimal health, who is able to resist both mental and physical setbacks no matter what they encounter, compared with those people who tend to unravel at the biological and emotional seams. These characteristics are control, predictability, and optimism.

When referring to control I don't mean being manipulative and controlling of other people. A healthy person is going to be in control of their own emotions, who can correctly and appropriately appraise their own emotional state, as well as that of others. They respond decisively and appropriately in the context of whatever is happening.

It is the person who collects information, who is open-minded; who provides themselves with the ability to predict what is likely to happen in the future. The inability to predict will give rise to perhaps the one emotion that will destroy relationships, interfere with your professional life, and erode your health more than any other emotion. And that emotion is fear.

In the professional setting it might be fear of failure, or of success, in learning something new, or accepting a promotion. In the context of relationships it might be not saying what needs to be said, or not taking steps to improve that relationship. Of course the incessant fear that goes on for a prolonged amount of time is going to result in activation of physiological pathways which will eventually erode your ability to fight disease.

Fear is the emotion of the future. It is perhaps the only emotion that is exclusively related not to the past or present, but rather to the future. In other words, you can only be afraid of something that has not happened. If it has already happened, you can be angry, disgusted, or sad, but not afraid. The reason fear is associated with the future is because we cannot predict what is going to happen next. If we know more we will fear less.

I am going to provide you with information that will be a very important part of staying well, because it will provide you with the understanding to make predictions. You will gain a better awareness of why some types of inflammatory symptoms are more likely to flare up at certain times as opposed to others, and then you can take the necessary precautions to avoid those situations. Or if not avoidable, by understanding how and why these outcomes occur, you begin to realize this is just a temporary setback, which can instill a sense of optimism that things will get back to normal, that you'll be back on track; the disease hasn't gotten worse.

Optimism is a word I'm going to use, however, not synonymously with positive thinking. Positive thinking is okay, but in excess it can sometimes be a very unhealthy coping style especially if it's used to obscure the bad thing that has happened. I'm using the word optimism the way that Dr. Marty Seligman did in characterizing the optimistic versus pessimistic explanatory style.

A healthy person, one who is likely to achieve a state of optimal health, can acknowledge that bad things happen; they won't deny it. However, they also recognize that this is not something that is permanent. This too shall eventually pass. They realize that it is a setback only in the context in which it has occurred, and they recognize that it doesn't have to permeate their entire life.

It might be something that is going to interfere with their professional development, but not relationships, or vice versa. They are people who do not personalize. They recognize that while they might have contributed to the outcome, there were outside factors that they had no control over that also played a role. So when I use the word optimism I'm referring to the optimistic explanatory style which means you don't personalize, you don't recognize events as being permanent, and they are not all pervasive.

These are the things that characterize those people who remain healthy. These are the things that you should be striving towards—learning ways to take control over your own emotions, and your overall health, gaining knowledge that helps you to predict, thereby lessening fear, and finally, learning how you can achieve that feeling of optimism.

A few years ago I was giving a presentation on how to achieve optimal health. I spent most of the day speaking about things that people can do, not only about the immune system but also heart health and mental health. At the end a woman said, "Dr. Hall, this has been very interesting. You have validated a lot of the things that I was already aware of. However, you failed to answer the one question that I need answered in order to make the changes that will get me to point of health that I am trying to achieve." I said, "What is your question?" She said, "I know what to do, so why don't I do it?"

That is the question and it remains unanswered. There is a multibillion dollar industry driven by the sale of self-help books and materials, and it seems every year there is a new expert touting a new formula, the secret that will enable you to achieve the state of optimal health. Why do people continue to spend millions of dollars every year for something new if that magical intervention was so wonderful? Why isn't it working? Why do people continue going back and getting more?

I believe the reason is that people don't have the motivation to act on the information they have available to them. The person who is going to achieve the state of health they desire is not the person with the most knowledge. It's not the person who has shelves full of books on nutrition or has an understanding of how the immune system works. No, it is the person who has the motivation to apply that information.

There are two additional questions she could have asked. I know what to do, so why can't I do it, which of course deals with the physiological changes, the barriers a person might have. If you have an immune gene which happens to leave you vulnerable to certain infections, there may not be a lot you can do about that. Obviously if you suffer from chronic fatigue or a metabolic disorder, there would be physical impediments that are definitely going to limit your options.

I am not going to tell you how you can make that disease disappear, that is really not what we are interested in doing. It is unrealistic to think you can make the disease disappear or that you can correct the genetic mutation, the abnormality, or the metabolic sequences going on in your body that give rise to disease.

What is realistic and what we really want to do is to better manage the symptoms. All of the information I am presenting about mobilizing your immune system and keeping it optimal, is designed to help you to keep those symptoms from interfering with life, liberty, and happiness. That first question—I know what to do so why can't I do it?—addresses the more identifiable obstacles that may be keeping the person from doing the things they know they ought to be doing. The other question to ask is, "I know what to do so why *won't* I do it? This second question addresses the motivational-side of the equation.

This information is useless if you can't motivate yourself to follow through and apply it. The most important bit of advice I can give is to be very careful how you define success, especially in the context of health. Realize that optimal health is not the absence of disease. We all have aches and pains, we all have abnormalities, or at least most of us do, and there's probably not a lot you can do about it.

I have permanent rheumatoid arthritis in my right thumb courtesy of a six foot alligator who one summer almost took my hand off. As a student in high school and college, I had a summer job at a tourist attraction called the Black Hills Reptile Gardens in South Dakota. During the 1960s I was their chief alligator wrestler, and it happened during a show when I jumped on the alligator's back and he was able to get his mouth secured around my hand before I had an opportunity to get my hands around his mouth and secure him.

There's not much I can do about it, and in cold weather it tends to drive me nuts. Don't feel sorry for me, the discomfort reminds me of those wonderful summers as a teenager when I lived on a cot in the basement, with essentially no adult supervision, nearly 2,000 miles from my home in Massachusetts. I have wonderful memories that occur every time I feel that pain and discomfort.

However, it is a reminder that we all have made mistakes, bad choices, or perhaps endured injury during sports, and as a result we pay the price for the rest of our lives. There is nothing I can do about the problem itself, but what I can do is take control over the symptoms. I have learned to predict what circumstances are likely to make those symptoms worse and that is the time when I will consume an anti-inflammatory diet. I will go out of my way to avoid those things that might make the symptoms even more difficult to deal with.

If you have rheumatoid arthritis or any type of illness, the objective should never be to get rid of the disease, in part, because that is unrealistic. If you define success as getting rid of the illness, you'll never know if you really succeeded. You will most likely be nagged with the thought that it is only a temporary state of remission waiting to rear its ugly clinical head when you might least expect it. Instead, your goal should be to better manage the symptoms. I believe that's all any of us is really interested in.

Regardless of whatever disease I may get: cancer, heart disease, small pox; I just don't want it to kill me. I don't want it to shorten my lifespan by a single millisecond. I don't want it to interfere with my productivity, nor my capacity for pleasure. If that disease wants to hangout in my body as long as it leaves me alone I'm perfectly willing to have a commensurate relationship with it. You leave me alone, I'll leave you alone, and we'll both be fine.

Obviously, I'm being facetious and if I were diagnosed with small pox or cancer I'd be devastated just like anyone else. I would hope that after I got over the initial shock, I would come out of my depression and start doing what I am telling you to do, and that is take steps to control the symptoms. We must also realize there are factors that you can't control. There are too many factors such as your genetic blueprint, environmental circumstances and other biological considerations, that might exacerbate the illness, and over which you have no direct control.

You don't want to focus on those things. You don't want to have as a goal something that you have limited control over. Instead you need to define success as making progress towards a worthwhile goal, which in this particular case is a state of optimal health. Make sure that the steps you take are ones that define your progress in ways that you have complete control over it.

I'll give you an example of how I do this. One of my favorite pastimes is being on the water in human-powered boats, kayaks, small sail boats, canoes. There's an organization called Water Tribe, which is comprised of an eclectic group of people who come together from various countries: Russia, New Zealand, England, and all over America; to participate in what has been identified as one of the most extreme endurance races on the planet. The short races are 300 miles in length; the premier event is 1,250 miles.

When I stand on the beach at the beginning of that 1,200 mile race with my kayak a few feet away there is no way that my goal is going to be getting to the finish. It is going to take me close to a month before I get there, it's too far off. I have the attention span of a four-year old. There's no way I can concentrate on something that is that far away.

Neither is my goal to get to the first checkpoint by a certain time. Nor is it to cover a certain distance per day. I can't control that. I have no way of controlling the weather, I don't know if I'm going to be facing gale force headwinds that are going to slow me to a crawl, I don't know when a piece of critical equipment is going to fail, or when I'm going to encounter a tide that is going against me. I'm not going to define a goal in a manner that's going to be influenced mostly by factors I have no control over.

My goal in these races is always to make forward progress and a minimum of 18 hours a day. One time I was about 3 miles out in the Atlantic Ocean, in the middle of the night when a critical piece of equipment failed. I had to spend the entire next day walking around different marinas searching for the parts and then the use the machine shop so I could make the necessary repairs. I counted that as making forward progress towards my goal. I didn't get a meter closer to my destination, but I counted that as making forward progress because it was something that had to be done.

It doesn't matter how fast I am going because my goal is defined in a way that's independent of speed and distance. Furthermore, I am automatically making progress with the passing of each minute. In 2006, at the start of the inaugural event called the Ultimate Florida Challenge, there were 50 people on the beach. Seven of us finished.

Among the ones who didn't finish were many who had objectives and goals framed in terms of speed and distance which they couldn't control. When they realized at the end of the day they had failed to achieve the goal they became despondent. They started focusing on other things that went wrong. It zapped their motivation and they started looking for excuses to drop out.

In the context of health your goal should not be to lose weight. Your goal should be to exercise 30 minutes every day because you have control over that. Your goal should be to limit the number of calories you take in each day because you have control over that. As a result of doing those things, by taking control over the things you can, losing weight will be the reward.

What are some of the things that you can control in the context of your immune system? What are some of the things that you can do to make sure that you stay in that preclinical phase after you've been exposed to something? First of all you might be wondering why I am not saying you should take steps to avoid exposure in the first place. Wouldn't that be better?

Absolutely not. First of all, it is unrealistic. How on earth are you going to avoid exposure to microbes and still succeed in life? Second, you don't want to do that. Use it or lose it is a phrase that applies not only to muscle physiology; it applies to your immune system as well. Your immune system needs to have a workout every now and then.

Of course we don't want exposure to things like anthrax or the Ebola virus. I'm referring to the microbes we are exposed to on a regular basis, microbes we want protection against. Exposure to those microbes provides you with the ability to build up memory cells which are going to protect you later on. In some instances they may protect you for the rest of your life.

When you are vaccinated against a microbe you are being treated with the exposure to the attenuated form of, for example the virus. By having the memory cells produced in response to that virus when your body is exposed to the live fully virulent wild form they can go into action very, very quickly and in most instances will keep you completely in that preclinical phase. You won't even know you were exposed, and if you do experience symptoms they will be a fraction of what they would have been without that exposure through the vaccine.

Of course we get exposure to the wild forms of microbes as well, and when those memory cells are formed the probability that you will succumb to symptoms upon subsequent exposure is significantly reduced. If you want to raise a really sickly child or animal take that individual at a very early age and raise it in a sterile environment. Filter all of the air going into the enclosure, sterilize the food, the water, and by the time that individual is a year you will see that person or that animal is going to be more susceptible to infection than those allowed to experience contact with microbial organisms.

This is because the immune system has had minimal stimulation or none at all. It has failed to produce any memory cells that will protect against microorganisms later in life. Shielding yourself from microbes is not only unrealistic; it is something you don't really want to be doing unless it is something capable of overwhelming your immune system.

Very interesting studies have been published over the years showing that children who live on farms are in contact with animals and children who go to daycare are exposed to the germs carried by other children and both are far less likely to develop asthma and allergies. They are healthier overall than children who are scrubbed squeaky clean every single day and whose parents take dramatic steps to minimize their exposure to pathogens. Since it's not practical to control and eliminate the circumstances that might lead to exposure to viruses and bacteria, then what do you have control over?

The symptoms that might arise, that's what you have control over. To accomplish that objective you need to have a basic understanding of the immune system and how it works. The immune system is comprised of two overlapping parts. One in particular plays a critical role in keeping you from experiencing symptoms. It happens to be called the innate immune system.

When the going gets really tough and this branch of the immune system is unable to counter the microbial onslaught, that's when the second branch is brought in to play: the highly specialized part of the immune system referred to as adaptive immunity. When that happens chemicals that make you feel awful are released in very large amounts. The chemicals that are required to mobilize that very skilled part of your immune system are the same ones that act in the brain to sap your motivation, to leave you feeling lethargic, flat on your back, unable to muster up the desire to do much of anything, even those things that would normally give rise to pleasure.

I want to point out that I will be sacrificing a certain degree of accuracy for the sake of clarity. For example I've already mentioned the innate versus the adaptive immune system, implying that they are separate entities, which is something I am doing so you can understand the role of each. In reality we're talking about one large system. There is constant communication between the two and all other components are interacting with each other.

For now, I'll start with the innate immune system which is comprised of physical barriers, cells, as well as the chemicals those cells produce. The innate immune system has a very large advantage which is that it is basically ready to go. Very little priming is required and what little is needed takes place in a matter of hours. That is not true of the adaptive immune system comprised mostly of T-cells and B-cells.

They have to be stimulated before undergoing various stages of maturation. It may require three to five days before you have adequate antibody titers to help protect you from whatever gave rise to their production. Not only that, the innate immune system is relatively nonspecific. It doesn't care what comes into the body.

Physical barriers will block any microbe that is likely to enter the body while the macrophages and monocytes are just as likely to reach out and grab influenza A, and then a moment later reach out and grab rhinovirus or the organism that causes tetanus. In other words they have no standards. If it doesn't belong in the body, if it doesn't have your HLA type or part of the major histocompatibility complex, then it's fair game for destruction. Your major histocompatibility complex is your chemical signature, a microscopic signature that identifies each cell as belonging to you.

That is absolutely not true of lymphocytes called T-cells and B-cells. These cells are specific, ones that protect you against influenza A will offer little if any protection against influenza B. That gives them a huge advantage. You can think of the adaptive immune system, the T lymphocytes and the B lymphocytes, as the equivalent of military Special Forces. They are trained to do one specific job and they do it extraordinarily well.

When you bring in the T and B-cells there's a very high likelihood of getting rid of those microbes. There is a price to pay because the chemical signals that come from other parts of the body to activate those T and B-cells are, as I noted before, the ones that make you feel lousy. The fevers, the aches, the pain, the lack of motivation, the lethargy are not caused directly by the virus.

Those symptoms are caused by your own activated immune system, something I'll be elaborating upon later.

If your main objective is to stay in the preclinical phase free of annoying symptoms, then your main objective is to keep from having to activate those T and B-cells. You need to takes steps to make sure that the innate immune system can get the job done very quickly in order to avoid the need to bring in the specialists. Before we continue I want to emphasize the importance of providing the basic ingredients so your immune system has a good foundation. Consider the foods and nutrition that you need to make sure your overall state of health is ready to join with fine-tuning your immune system.

Nutrition and Your Immune System

What are the micronutrients that you need to have in your body to provide an overall state of optimal immunity so that when you need that immune system, it's able to perform in the way that you want it to? There are certain nutrients which have the potential to alleviate the symptoms associated with an infection, especially vitamin A.

When Vitamin A was first being characterized it was often referred to as the anti-infection vitamin. It optimizes white cell function, which is what lymphocytes are, and it maintains the mucosal tissues. The mucous membranes provide a gooey solution which tends to trap pathogens, keeping them from getting elsewhere into the body and enabling the adjacent immune cells to neutralize it before it can cause symptoms. Vitamin A is necessary to maintain those mucous membranes. Carrots, spinach, kale, Brussels sprouts, apricots, mango, cantaloupe and cayenne are all very good sources of vitamin A.

Vitamin C has several different roles to play. You need it to maintain collagen, the foundation of the skin. It's also anti-inflammatory and serves as an antioxidant. You especially need vitamin C to maintain the integrity of your phagocytic cells. These are the so-called Pac-Men of the immune system, which mobilize, wrap their membrane around the virus, and ingest it. You need vitamin C in order to make sure those cells are able to work optimally. Papaya, red bell peppers, broccoli, oranges, cantaloupe and kale are excellent sources of vitamin C.

Copper is a mineral that you need to reduce free radicals. Free radicals will wreak havoc in your body if you have too many so that the body's natural systems to neutralize them are overwhelmed. Turnips, spinach, kale, eggplant, tomatoes, cashews, ginger root and beans are excellent sources of copper. You need selenium, as well, in order to protect cells from oxidative stress. Asparagus, spinach, cod, shrimp, salmon, turkey, barley and chicken are very good sources of selenium.

Zinc is found to improve the functioning of white cells which you need to mobilize your immune system. They also decrease immunoglobulin E-mediated histamine release, responsible for some of the pain and discomfort associated with the inflammation surrounding the elimination of a pathogen. Summer squash, asparagus, broccoli, green peas and collard greens are good sources of zinc.

In the average American diet, a lot of people don't get enough Omega-3 fatty acids, which play multiple roles within the body. Recent studies have shown that Omega-3 fatty acids are an antioxidant as well as a powerful anti-inflammatory factor able to reduce the production of the chemicals responsible for the pain and discomfort associated with inflammation. When Omega-3 is administered to people suffering from mild, traumatic brain injury, it seems to have efficacy in improving their condition as well. Fish is a very good source of Omega-3s, especially salmon, halibut, shrimp and scallops. Non-animal sources include flax seeds, walnuts, broccoli, cauliflower, tofu and soybeans.

Bromelain is an ingredient necessary to maintain the mucolytic and anti-inflammatory processes in the body. Pineapple is a good source of that. Capsaicin is the spice people use to add a little pizazz to food. It'll clear your sinuses. It'll promote drainage and relieve pain. Cayenne pepper is a good source of capsaicin.

Probiotics have also been found to optimize the immune system. Probiotics are sources of bacteria. Lactobacillus is a probiotic that you need in certain body environments to maintain optimal health. Yogurt, cottage cheese, aged cheese, miso, pickles and wine are good sources of probiotics.

These are the things that can help mobilize your immune system in fighting an infection. While inflammation is the process that enables you to contain the infectious agent and keep it from spreading around the body, at the same time, too much inflammation can cause major problems. Inflammation is not only a process that is essential if you want to stay healthy, but inflammation can sometimes turn against you and become the cause of a problem.

If you were like I was, bitten by an alligator, or perhaps there was a car accident or a sports injury, afterwards there can be problems with inflammation stemming from that injury. This is sometimes referred to as sterile inflammation. Sterile, because there are no bacteria or viruses involved. The symptoms associated with this inflammation range from simply annoying to excruciatingly painful.

There are things that you can do to bring down sterile inflammation. Fruits and vegetables such as apples and onions contain quercetin and have the potential of alleviating symptoms, especially those of allergic rhinitis. This is the type of allergy you experience when you suffer from exposure to tree pollen or ragweed, which are very common allergens in America. Extra-virgin olive oil, flax seeds, rosemary, salmon, halibut, and spirulina all have the potential to alleviate those symptoms as well.

It is not just a matter of adding things to your diet in order to stay well. There are certain things you want to avoid such as dairy products. Dairy contains milk, a wonderful source of protein, but it is animal protein, the cow's protein, which sometimes can trigger mild inflammation and allergic type symptoms in us. You may find yourself clearing your throat more. If you have rhinitis and inflammation involving the upper respiratory pathways, you don't want anything that's going to stimulate extra mucous. Other things that you might want to cut back on or avoid include yeast products, such as bread, refined sugars and alcohol, artificial food additives, as well as salts. Some of the things you can do to optimize your system and better manage the symptoms include: steam inhalation, drinking hot teas such as ginger and consuming broth-based soups, spicy foods, horseradish and hot peppers.

Saline-based nasal washes can be beneficial for some people as well as plant-based supplements containing Sinupret, quercetin, and bromelain. Consume a well-balanced diet with adequate Omega-3 fatty acids, and cut back on Omega-6s. Omega-3 fatty acids are anti-inflammatory. Omega-6 fatty acids are pro-inflammatory.

The average American diet provides a person with too little Omega-3s and too many Omega-6s, which is one of the reasons Dean Ornish and Dr. Andrew Weil have characterized the average American diet as being pro-inflammatory. Other beneficial supplements include Vitamin A and spirulina, which is a chlorophyll-rich algae capable of increasing immunoglobulin A (IgA). IgA is the antibody referred to as the anti-infection antibody.

Take steps to reduce exposure to environmental and known food allergens, things that might stimulate an allergic reaction, where the symptoms would overlap with those associated with rhinitis. Those are the things that you ought to be doing all the time in order to maintain a good foundation.

Let's address the specific components of the innate immune system and some additional things you can do to make sure it works for you when you need it. The nonspecific branch of the immune system, also called the innate immune system, is comprised first and foremost of physical barriers, the most important of which is the outer waterproof covering, the skin that we are all squeezed into. There is no question that the skin is a physical barrier. If you visit any burn unit and you will quickly learn just how important our skin really is. When the skin becomes compromised as will occur in severe burn patients, the biggest problem is infection. There is no longer a barrier to keep swarms of bacteria from getting in and burn victims often succumb to overwhelming systemic infection or sepsis.

Along with the skin as our first barrier, there are dynamic processes going on as well. For example, natural antibiotics are being produced by epithelial cells within the skin and by neutrophils and other cell types throughout the body. These natural antibiotics, called defensins and cathelicidins, help to neutralize bacteria within the body.

A very large number of bacteria exist on your skin, in a commensurate relationship with you. These bacteria are there, and able to compete with harmful bacteria that try to invade the body. To underscore just how important it is to maintain the integrity of these bacteria on the skin, we can look to some recent research published on diabetic mice, often used as a model of the human equivalent his disease.

People with diabetes have difficulty recovering from external injuries. It takes a long time for an injury to heal. Part of the reason is the interruption of circulation of blood into the area, and now this study indicates it is related to the bacterial flora which normally resides on the skin.

It was found that the diabetic mice had about 40 times the amount of bacteria on their skin, compared with the non-diabetic animals. However, they had very few varieties of bacteria which correlates with their inability to mount an adequate response when engaged in wound healing. It is not yet clear exactly how all of this fits together, but it certainly suggests a very important role for these bacteria that normally reside on the skin.

There's a quantum leap between the laboratory, where animals are studied, and the human clinic. You have to be very careful when interpreting the data that have been collected as a part of a well-controlled laboratory study and then applying that knowledge in the context of human illness.

We have learned so much about the human condition through these types of experiments and while we may need to adjust our ultimate interpretation of these results, the recent research is strongly suggesting the potential for an expanded role of bacteria on the skin. You must have the right amount and the right variety of bacteria in order to maintain the integrity of your physical barriers, your skin.

That would be a very strong reason to avoid washing your hands obsessively in antibiotic soaps, thereby weakening this barrier. I say this regarding normal circumstances because today we are living under abnormal ones with the possibility of exposure to new and highly infectious superbugs against which antibiotics are ineffective. There are some people who do need to take extra precautions, for example, people working in hospital settings, where they might have undue exposure to microbes. Extra precautions are necessary to protect themselves as well as their patients.

If you work with very young children, you may realize that young kids often have no personal hygiene. Children are vectors of disease, so you do need to take extra precautions.

When my youngest grandchild has a cold and I pick him up, he takes great delight huffing, sneezing, then wiping his nose with his hand and smearing it on Grandpa's face. I know what he's doing.

At the subconscious level, he is aware that my immune system, because of age is beginning to wane. He's increasing my exposure to microbes in order to hasten my demise so he can get his hands on my resources. Actually, I probably did the same thing to my grandparents and just as the medieval wheel of fortune symbolized, what goes around, comes around.

I am completely serious about the part where exposure to young children does increase the probability that you're going to come in contact with microbes. Under those circumstances you do need to take extra precautions to remain in that preclinical phase and to stay well. But under normal circumstances, if you do not work in an environment where you have undo exposure to bacteria and viruses, leave the microbiota, that natural bacterial layer that you have on your skin alone. Let them do their job. Don't put selective pressure on them forcing them to turn into superbugs, which will later become resistant to those antimicrobial soaps and at a time when you may need them under circumstances when your immune system may not be up to the task.

Remember the wonder drugs: penicillin, tetracycline, and ampicillin? They were so effective in their day in fighting large numbers and different species of bacteria. Many of them are now practically useless, largely because of the widespread use of antibiotics in the meat and poultry industry and because they have been prescribed as placebos.

One of the most common placebos administered to patients is an antibiotic. So, we've applied selective pressure, forcing the most resistant ones to survive. Because bacteria proliferate so quickly, they have evolved into forms that are now completely resistant to many antibiotics that we have available.

The skin is not the only barrier. Others are comprised of secretions—the mucous secretions in the nasal passages, saliva in the oral cavity, secretions which line the respiratory tree, as well as the gastrointestinal tract. In the nasal passages, these secretions help to create a most inhospitable environment for a lot of microbes.

When bacteria get in there, they have to run a gauntlet. They have to get through all of this sticky stuff, which is going to bog them down. They have to dodge the hair cells. That is one of the reasons why I recommend that if you absolutely have to pick your nose, use your left index finger, not your right. Don't use the hand that you just shook hands with, the one you opened the door with, and then take that finger and shove that virus you were exposed to right past the mucous secretions, past the hair cells, into the area where it wants to be.

Make it work. Use your left hand, not the hand you used to open doors, to sign your name at the hotel registration desk, to shake hands with people. The obvious corollary of that is to keep your hands away from your face in the first place. That is probably the best thing you can do to protect yourself from infection against any sort of flu or cold.

But how many people are going to be able to consciously do that? We put our hands up to our eyes, our nose, and our mouth multiple times throughout the day. One of the things that we can do is consciously train ourselves to use our left hands more, instead of the right. Though I was being facetious when I talked about which hand is best for picking your nose, I am also completely serious. We know it is best to avoid putting the hand that is most likely to come into contact with microbes near those regions where the microbe is able to take hold and enter your body.

Through practice, you can actually change habits. Habits form only through repetition. There is nothing to stop you from creating a new repertoire of habits, one that is going to be conducive to keeping you in that healthy state.

Within these secretions, there are specialized chemicals. One of the most important is referred to as immunoglobulin A, not to be confused with vitamin A, which is a nutrient. Immunoglobulin A is sometimes referred to as secretory IgA because it's chemically fortified to survive in this very harsh environment. When it sticks to a microbe, it weakens it, rendering it more susceptible to destruction by macrophages.

There are other chemicals that contribute as well, ones that we refer to as pro-inflammatory cytokines. These help to mobilize our natural defenses so that you can nip the infection in the bud and get rid of it before it gets past the barrier. This is the entry point for most microbes. It's very rare when something enters the body through the skin. Most microbes enter the body through the respiratory tree or we put things into our mouths. That's why it is so important to take care of this environment.

I'd like to expand upon our earlier discussion of the nutrients critical to maintaining the integrity of these particular barriers. One of the things that you might be asking is, exactly how much vitamin A? How much vitamin C? How much of these nutrients do we actually need in order to stay well?

That is hard to say exactly, but here is what you need to keep in mind as you decide for yourself how much of a particular nutrient you might need. If you were to draw a schematic of a human body, running down the center would be a hollow tube. It begins at the mouth. It ends at the anus. Everything that is inside that tube is technically outside the body. It is not inside the body until it crosses the membrane.

There are a lot of things that will interfere with the absorption of nutrients as well as viruses and bacteria. If you have any type of inflammation associated with the upper part of the small intestine where most micronutrients enter the body, that inflammation will interfere with the absorption. Even though you may be ingesting, let's say 100% of the vitamin A that you need to have in your system, if there are circumstances going on in your GI system resulting in only perhaps 50% of that vitamin A getting absorbed, then you need to ingest more. You need to start out with more in order to end up having available to the cells, what is actually needed.

That applies to every vitamin. If you are an athlete, realize there is not enough blood in the circulatory system to fill every capillary bed simultaneously. Blood has to be diverted. When a person is exercising, the blood is diverted from the gastrointestinal system to the muscles that are being used.

If there is not enough blood circulating through the capillary beds that line the small intestine, then food that is ingested right after exercise is not going to be absorbed very well. It's not going to be taken up into the body as it could be if ingested at a later time. There are some foods that are very sticky. Soluble fiber, for example, that bowl of oatmeal you might eat in the morning, sticks to things, including vitamins. So even though you may start out with a large amount, just what you need to stay healthy, if you are taking that vitamin or eating that source of vitamin with a lot of fiber, then you need to take into account that a smaller percentage than what you started with is actually getting into the body across those membranes.

There are plenty of books and websites that will tell you what the average person needs in order to remain healthy. There are nutritional associations, the FDA, the USDA, government agencies that are monitoring the health of people. They are looking at people's eating habits and coming up with recommendations of how much of different nutrients a person needs on average to stay healthy.

Use that as a starting point, as a way to experiment with your body and see what you need in order to remain healthy. If you have any type of medical condition and you believe that nutrients are a factor, that either you are missing something in your diet, or perhaps by adding more of something, you might be able to better deal with the symptoms, then my recommendation is to consult with a registered dietician, one who has experience working with the medical condition that you are concerned about, and follow their advice. When you have an illness of any type, the rules change, and what you would predict based upon a well-controlled laboratory study is not always the way it works when you have a system that is broken, when you have any type of clinical condition.

Though we have been discussing the nutrients that needed to stay healthy and maintain optimal immunity, I have not yet mentioned the most important one of all. I wanted to save that and give it more time because of its importance. And that is water, hydration.

In the average person, 60 to 70 percent of their body weight is going to be comprised of water, most of which is inside the cells. It's not in the bloodstream. It's not in the cerebral spinal fluid. It's in their cells. It's absolutely critical that hydration be in the proper range in different compartments within your body so that there is sufficient fluidity to maintain electrolyte balance, to enable the membranes to have the ingredients they need for substrates that are going to build cytokines and antibodies to get in and for the end product, the defensins, the cathelicidins, the natural antibiotics, to get out.

Let's talk about hydration and some of the things that can affect it. One of the ways that stress impacts your body is by causing your mouth to dry up. You've all experienced it, I'm sure. Perhaps, when you were in first grade and the teacher asked you to come to the front of the room and tell everyone where you went on your summer holiday. Public speaking is a major stressor for a lot of people, at least before they become accustomed to it. Your mouth probably became so dry you couldn't even tell people what your name was.

That's because of activation of a branch of the nervous system called the sympathetic nervous system. The main chemical produced is called epinephrine, which is not only capable of down-regulating the immune system but at the same time, it tends to trigger dehydration. Epinephrine is the same chemical that is put into a syringe referred to as an EpiPen.

People who are highly susceptible to the toxin in bee venom, for example, will often carry an EpiPen, so if they get stung by a bee, they almost immediately inject that epinephrine into themselves in order to suppress their immune system to prevent an overzealous, inflammatory response referred to as anaphylaxis. If they go into anaphylactic shock, they could very well die. That's why it's so critical. This is the same epinephrine that is being produced when your sympathetic nervous system becomes activated, and that happens when you find yourself under stress.

In order for that immunoglobulin A and the other chemicals found in saliva and those mucous secretions to bathe the tongue, the lips, the gums, there has to be a certain amount of hydration. Obviously, if the sympathetic nervous system is decreasing salivation, then the bioavailability of these critical chemicals to remain in that preclinical phase, are not going to be there. Stress is a shift from building to breaking things down. In biochemical terms, we would call it a switch from anabolism to catabolism. The rationale is quite logical. Why build for the future if there is going to be no future?

Digesting food is all about the future. Digesting food, especially protein, is like going to the hardware store and buying building materials in order to undertake a construction project. The amino acids that you ingest in meat, as well as legumes, the vegetable source of protein are the building blocks for the receptors that are going to be built, for muscles, for many hormones. So that is building. Salivation is the first step in digestion. That's going to be inhibited as well as the body switches to breaking things down, mobilizing resources that are needed.

It's one of the reasons why people do become more susceptible to infections during times of stress, going through a divorce or the night before a major exam. In part, this is because their immune system is being compromised. They have increased exposure. They lack the ingredients that are necessary to keep the microbe from getting into the body. At the same time, the cells are not able to work as efficiently.

I'll jump ahead and tell you right now that anything that you do to alleviate the stress in your life is going to benefit your immune system. As you listen as I continue this discussion, always keep that in mind. Taking steps to reduce stress is not just a matter of feeling more relaxed and calm, getting better sleep. There's a critical link between stress and the immune system.

In order to underscore just how important these barriers are, I'll introduce you to a group of people who many would consider some of the healthiest on the planet, ultra-marathoners. These are people who begin the day by swimming several miles in the open ocean, then hop on their bicycles and ride over 100 miles before putting on their running shoes and completing a full marathon. They do that all in the same day. If it's part of the premier event, the Ironman Competition, they are doing it in the mountains of Hawaii, and there is absolutely no question from a cardiovascular standpoint, these people are second to none.

Dr. Ken Cooper, who founded the Aerobic Institute in Dallas, Texas, would give them five gold stars for building their cardiovascular fitness. From a mental toughness standpoint, these people are absolutely extraordinary. The ability to get out there and train, often in very inhospitable conditions, takes a huge amount of willpower. I have the utmost respect for these athletes.

From an immune system standpoint, these extreme athletes are train wrecks, very sickly, prone to one upper respiratory infection after another, especially during the two weeks following the event. There are two reasons, and both involve the oral cavity. They have increased exposure to microbes, and at the same time, their immune system is diminished. In other words, they are experiencing the perfect immunologic storm.

Why do they have increased exposure? It is not because somebody ran through the streets of Boston, or sprayed the course with aerosol-containing viruses. Remember, I told you that something is not in the body, yet. The cells are not exposed until that microbe crosses the membranes.

Dehydration diminishes the ability of the mucous secretions, these outer membranes that are so critically important, to work optimally. It is not increased exposure to the microbe in the external environment; it is increased exposure in the internal environment, within the body. Normally, that microbe would stay within the nasal passages or be destroyed in the GI system.

In the same way that nutrients have to get into the body, viruses and bacteria also have to get into the body and pass through the membrane. Because of dehydration, the ultra-marathoner's susceptibility and exposure is greater. And let's face it, if you are going to be competitive in one of these events, there is no way you can stop and remain properly hydrated. The best an athlete will do is grab a cup of water from somebody standing there who hands it to them on the side of the road, take a swig, toss it into the bushes, and without even breaking stride, keep going.

Dehydration ensures that the secretions that normally provide the obstacle course for viruses to negotiate before they can get into the body are basically going to be dried up. It's very interesting to note that the athletes who are very competitive, the ones who normally win, are the ones who are most vulnerable to upper respiratory infections, not the people who just want to get the t-shirt and say I did this. The more competitive folks will turn on the afterburners, especially during the final miles. They switch from aerobic to anaerobic metabolism, and in order to take in enough oxygen to keep going, they have no choice but to suck that air directly into their lungs, bypassing all of these barriers. Of course, even if they were to breathe through their nose, it's probably not going to do them any good because everything is dried up.

By the way, if you are working in an environment where someone happens to be coughing and sneezing, or if you travel a lot, and you are breathing recycled air in airplanes, then one thing you can do to stay well is to make sure you do breathe through your nose, not through your mouth. Stay hydrated. Make sure you drink plenty of water. It may be difficult to keep track of, but if you can consciously make yourself aware of it and remind yourself to do it as often as possible, that will give you a huge advantage and the increased likelihood that you will stay in that preclinical phase.

The things that we do routinely without thinking about them are habits. Many people don't know whether they breathe through their nose or their mouth most of the time. One of the most effective ways of training yourself is to provide feedback for yourself. In other words, pay attention to it.

Keep track, and start consciously thinking, am I breathing through my nose or my mouth? If you are breathing through your mouth, then practice breathing through your nose. You're going to add another layer of filtration, decreasing the likelihood that you will be exposed to the microbes.

Stress and Immunity

There are different types of stress. Somatic stress, which is what I'm referring to now, is physical trauma to the body. It's what happens when you're in a car accident and you injure yourself. It's what happens when you put excessive demands on your body. You are breaking down muscle tissue, which has to be rebuilt. This type of exercise is a somatic stressor which these athletes are subjecting themselves voluntarily.

Psychogenic stress is the anticipation of trauma to the body. It's the type of stress a person who is worried about not performing well at work. It's that fear of failure that cripples a musician, keeps them from being able to play effectively in the orchestra. It's that anticipation of trauma, especially when you don't have control. You can't predict when it's going to be over. You lack any sense of optimism that things will ever get better. That is the type of stress that I think most of us are familiar with.

Both somatic and psychogenic stress will result in much of the same chemistry that can impair the immune system, your memory, as well as other critical functions in the body. And it turns out, the same chemical in the body that is able to down-regulate the immune system under stress, is the one that you produce to provide yourself with energy. It's called cortisol, and is produced by the adrenal glands.

Cortisol belongs to a family of chemicals called glucocorticoids. One of their primary missions in life is to provide glucose. When you run out of stored energy in the form of glycogen, the cortisol will start converting certain amino acids, the foundation of protein, into glucose. In other words, during times of stress, cortisol will put pennies into your pocket in order to fuel what Dr. Walter Cannon would have referred to as the fight-flight response.

A small amount of cortisol isn't going to be a problem. In fact, it stimulates the immune system and provides it with the energy it needs when fighting off an infection. However, when that cortisol becomes elevated for an extended period of time, as it would during the training or during the event, it's now part of the process whereby construction projects are shut down in order to make sure you survive the moment.

Let's break things down. Let's mobilize the energy that we have within the body to make sure it's available as you extricate yourself from this crisis. That includes the immune system. Who cares if your immune system becomes suppressed during times of stress? So what if you are more susceptible to influenza next season. If you're a cadaver, that is totally irrelevant.

Let's worry about fighting infection after the crisis is over. For now, we've got to survive. Don't worry about your T-cells and B-cells. Let it shut down. We'll rebuild it when the crisis is over.

The entire focus during an emergency is getting the energy to sustain that fight-flight response. The brain doesn't understand the difference. When a person is out there running, exercising excessively, as these ultra-marathoners do, the brain doesn't realize that they are doing it because they enjoy it. As far as the brain is concerned, they've been out there running miles every day in order to escape a pack of saber-toothed tigers. During the event, they must be bearing down very closely because now the athlete has turned on the afterburners. From a chemical standpoint, these people are experiencing a full-blown chemical stress response.

Cortisol happens to be anti-inflammatory. We have discussed inflammation in the context of fighting illness, and in the context of symptoms associated with rheumatoid arthritis, for example. Inflammation is a double-edged sword. If you don't have enough inflammation, you won't contain the infection. If you have too much inflammation, you'll suffer miserably.

It is the job of cortisol to make sure you don't have too much inflammation. It's the job of cortisol to push the immune system down when it goes up too high to keep it in that healthy mid-range. But if you have too much cortisol, as you would if you were stressed out excessively, which in effect is what these athletes are doing, it will push the immune system down to the point where it can no longer protect you. That is why these athletes are prone to upper respiratory infection.

Cortisol also shuts down the reproductive system. It inhibits luteinizing hormone, which will shut down ovulation in women and spermatogenesis in men; one of the reasons why these athletes can have difficulty getting pregnant. It makes perfect sense. Who wants to be saddled with a child if you're not going to be around to do the job of raising it.

It takes a very large number of calories to get a child from conception to parturition. If you need those calories to survive, if you need that energy right now to extricate yourself from an emergency, that's where those calories need to be. The stress response basically shuts down the entire reproductive system, including your libido.

The next time your significant other wants to go running all day with the attractive next door neighbor, let them go. They'll have neither the desire, nor the ability to do much else. Suggest they go off for the whole weekend, and that will enable you to have a fling yourself.

The reason I elaborated upon this population of ultra-marathoners is because we will come back and talk about them later on. The fact is, there are a lot of people who run multiple marathons every year, yet stay healthy. They do not succumb to repeated upper respiratory infection. They have figured out what to do. They have figured out what to do based upon a large amount of research sponsored by the sporting industry, Adidas, Nike, the makers of Gatorade, and Nestle who make power bars.

They don't want people lying on the couch recovering from infection. They want them wearing out their shoes, using their products, consuming their ingredients. It's a multi-billion-dollar a year industry and they have conducted a large amount of research to enable these athletes to stay healthy.

I firmly believe that by studying those people who subject themselves to the extremes, we can glean lessons that we can apply to ourselves. If a person who subjects himself to extreme stress voluntarily has figured out a way to maintain an optimal state of health, then why couldn't we do the same thing?

I am talking about those of us who are not exercising to that extreme, but with lesser degrees of stress or emotional upheaval. We all experience those everyday stressors, the interpersonal conflict, the problems with the infrastructure at work, the lousy reward system, deadlines, traffic and noise. Why not use the same techniques?

I am talking about the things that can be done with vitamin C, the way that you can manipulate carbohydrates in order to remain in that preclinical phase, despite the fact that you might have increased exposure to microbes. Let's say the microbe makes it you're your first line of barriers. The initial defenses are not successful in keeping it out. That's going to require mobilization of the phagocytic cells.

I told you that the definition of inflammation really is a process whereby the infection is contained. That means you want the immune system to go to the infection. You do not want the infection to go to the immune system. There are cells circulating in your bloodstream that have the potential of directly eating, or in immunology terms the word is phagocytosis, of ingesting that virus and thereby destroying it.

Neutrophils, a type of white cells circulating in the bloodstream are capable of doing this. Monocytes are another. Monocytes will get into the infected area and become transformed into what are called macrophages. These are the cell-eating or phagocytic cells. They are the equivalent of Pac-Man in the computer game that many people are familiar with, who mows through the obstacles.

They have to get there by circulating in the blood-stream. How does that happen? How does that neutro-phil that is circulating around in your carotid artery know that it needs to be down in your big toe after you have stepped on a piece of broken glass?

When you step on that glass, the injured cells almost immediately begin producing certain proteins. Some of those proteins, along with other factors being produced like prostaglandins, leukotrienes, and histamine, are going to separate from the endothelial cells making it possible for stuff to leak from the blood into the infected area.

Other chemicals are going to serve as chemical mag-nets. They are called chemokines. They get into the bloodstream, and when a neutrophil or monocyte catches a whiff of that chemical, they follow it down the concentration gradient, always taking the fork in the arterial road that will get it closer and closer to the highest amount of chemokines being produced. Obviously, the largest amount is going to be found at the site of the injury.

When the cell arrives, other chemicals that are part of the inflammatory response have opened up the gap between the cells lining the blood vessels. The cell gets in, fluid leaks in as well, and that is inflammation. The liquid stays there because all of that protein through osmosis keeps the fluid from leaking out. As a result, it swells up, the pressure is a trigger of pain exacerbated by the production of prostaglandins, and you have that all too familiar response. It might have happened when you twisted your ankle stepping off a stairway. It might have happened when you got an infection. But we're all familiar with the symptoms of inflammation.

In the context of fighting an infection, it is absolutely critical that you leave this process alone. Don't do anything unless it's absolutely imperative, unless there are going to be severe consequences, because anything that you do to slow down that type of inflammation is going to prolong the amount of time the infectious agent will stay in you. You might feel better, but if you can eliminate the cause of that inflammation as quickly as possible, that is what you want to be doing. In the long run, you will be better off.

The cell arrives, wraps its membrane around the virus, and encapsulates it. The membrane pinches off, and now the virus is floating inside this circular piece of membrane, which then combines with the cellular equivalent of a small bag containing meat tenderizers. Actually they are enzymes, which break down the virus. The virus is spit out, and you are well on your way to recovery.

There are two things that the phagocytic cells need, vitamin C and oxidative metabolites. Before I elaborate on why you need those, make sure that you create an environment that is conducive to these cells working optimally, which means things that you should not do. When they feel that soreness, that tenderness, many people will be tempted to go to the pharmacy and buy a cream containing synthetic glucocorticoid; names such as prednisone and hydrocortisone acetate. These are basically artificial forms of the natural cortisol your adrenals produce during stress, the cortisol which is anti-inflammatory.

They work almost immediately. Cortisol is a steroid; it is lipid or fat soluble and goes right through the skin. The pain relief is almost instantaneous, but there's a price to pay because what you're doing is blocking the inflammatory process. You are inhibiting the cells that are required now to get that microbe out of the way, and increasing the probability that it may go on and require activation of other parts of the immune system, which is going to result in the symptoms associated with the later stages. The whole purpose of this book is to learn about the things you can do to keep from advancing to the clinical phase of the infection.

Let's go back inside the phagocytic cell. As I mentioned previously, two things are needed, oxidative metabolites and vitamin C. Oxidative metabolites, for example, peroxide, superoxide and nitric oxide, are the byproducts of metabolism, specifically oxidative metabolism. The most common name that you are probably familiar with is free radicals.

Free radicals are very unstable molecules, and that is because they are missing an electron. Like everything in nature, they seek stability, and the way they get it is by stealing the electron from whatever happens to be nearby. If that free radical is being produced inside an activated macrophage, it's most likely going to steal the missing electron from the microbe that is now being brought inside, thereby hastening its destruction.

However, if you have excess free radicals, they may end up stealing the missing electron from the cell nucleus, altering its ability to maintain control over cell division. And yes, there is an association between excess free radicals and some forms of cancer. If that free radical is being formed inside the lining of your blood vessel wall, it may steal the electron from there setting the stage for atherosclerosis.

If it happens to be produced in the brain in association with the buildup of amyloid beta protein, those people who are diagnosed with Alzheimer's disease, it may steal the electron from an adjacent neuron hastening the dementia. Excess free radicals have indeed been linked with every category of serious human illness, cancer, Alzheimer's, and coronary arterial disease.

However, like everything pertaining to the immune system, they represent a double-edged sword. Don't demonize them. You have to have a certain number. Indeed, about 3% of the oxygen you take in with each and every breath is being converted into these oxidative metabolites.

There are some people who have a breakdown in their ability to produce these oxidative metabolites, and the resulting condition is referred to as chronic granulomatous disease. So you want to make sure that you have enough. Don't get carried away by taking lots of antioxidants. Only if you have excess free radicals do you really need to be worried about it. The fact is that most of us don't really need to worry about it at all.

The body produces enzymes, including dismutase and catalase, which help to neutralize the excess free radicals so they don't spill over and cause problems. Just about any diet that you consume is probably going to include quite a few natural antioxidants. Vitamins A, C, and E for example, will provide the missing electron. That's why they are referred to as antioxidants. The flavonoids in wine, as well as in tea, along with the Omega-3 fatty acids serve in this capacity as well.

There are plenty of things out there that you're probably doing all the time that will help you to maintain a healthy balance of these oxidative metabolites. There are always exceptions to every rule. There are some people whose circumstances may result in their having too many of these free radicals. For example, a person who lives in a polluted environment, who smokes cigarettes, who inhales a lot of secondhand smoke, or who work around equipment that generates electromagnetic frequencies is likely to have more than their fair share of free radicals.

Other risk is found in people who eat a large amount of fatty foods. Fat requires oxygen in order to burn, so the metabolism of those foods is going to generate more of these oxidative metabolites. Under those circumstances, this person may need to get extra antioxidants in the diet. Always, the best way to do this is to eat more of those foods that are rich in vitamins A, C, and E. Eat more fish or fish oil that contains the Omega-3 fatty acids.

Under some circumstances, you may not be able to get what you need by eating whole foods. If you spend a lot of time at 30,000 feet in airplanes logging 100,000 miles every year as a member of your frequent flyer club, then it is highly unlikely as you dash from terminal A to terminal D at a large metropolitan airport that you're going to be able to eat healthfully.

Living on a restricted income may also be a factor requiring supplements. A lot of elderly people cannot afford to eat the types of foods they need. Under those circumstances a supplement might be a good idea. If you can possibly do it the natural way, which is through whole foods, enabling your body to absorb just what it needs, that is the surest way of maintaining a state of optimal health and a healthy balance within your immune system.

Make sure that you've got what you need, but at the same time, don't exceed the threshold which could lead to serious health consequences. That applies certainly to vitamin C. Now, why exactly, is vitamin C important?

Inside the macrophage, as it's gobbling up the virus, there are free radicals being produced. I've already explained how these can help to speed up the demise of the virus. You don't want those free radicals spilling over and destroying mitochondria or ribosomes or some of the other things that are critical for the cell to function.

Vitamin C is water soluble. The fluid inside the cell is basically water. That's what cytosol is. You need something, an antioxidant that is water soluble inside the cell to soak up the extra free radicals so they don't impair the ability of that macrophage to do its job.

Now, the cell membrane is lipid. It's a fat. Vitamin C is not really going to do much in that environment. That's why you need vitamin E. Vitamin E is also a very powerful antioxidant. It's the one that's added to a lot of processed foods in order to keep the food from going rancid, from being oxidized.

You need the fat-soluble antioxidant to protect the cell membrane; you need the water-soluble vitamin C in order to protect the inside of the cell. Vitamin C is probably the most controversial nutrient out there. No one disagrees that you need it. The controversy is with respect to how much and in what form.

Some people argue that the amount recommended by the various nutritional associations: the FDA, a minimum of around 70 to 80 mg per day, is woefully inadequate. They base their arguments upon a claim made by Dr. Linus Pauling, a double Nobel Laureate, who proposed that when you first start feeling the symptoms of a cold, you need to be taking at least 1,000 mg of vitamin C per hour until the cold symptoms abate; a whopping dose.

The nutritionists of that era absolutely cringed, but what do you say to a Nobel Laureate, who has two Nobel prizes: one in biochemistry and one in peace. So they looked the other way and decided to call it water soluble. The excess will be flushed out of the body.

That began the largest uncontrolled experiment in the history of American medicine. Legions of people took Linus Pauling's advice and started taking huge doses; 500 mg, 1,000 mg, and even more, every single day. Some of them showed up in their doctors' offices with relatively mild symptoms, such as diarrhea and other GI upset.

But more serious conditions were showing up, too, such as scurvy, which is just the opposite of what you would expect. After all, a deficiency of vitamin C is the purported cause of scurvy, not an excess.

The type of scurvy that I'm referring to was first reported in babies born to mothers who took mega doses of vitamin C, and it makes perfect sense. Remember earlier I mentioned the idea of use it or lose it. I talked about how it applies to the immune system and to muscle physiology, and it also applies to vitamin C and other nutrients.

If a fetus is being provided with vitamin C in purified form on a silver platter, why do the cells need to crank up all that expensive enzymatic machinery to extract it from foods? They lack the ability, and when that child goes cold turkey, when the umbilical cord is cut, when that supply of purified vitamin C is cut off, they develop what is referred to in the medical literature as rebound scurvy.

Not long ago I was giving a lecture in New York City where a surgeon in the audience told about a patient who had stayed in the hospital several days longer than expected because he had developed scurvy. That was absolutely not on anybody's radar screen. Despite the fact that the dieticians in the hospital were making sure that all the patients got a well-balanced meal, it turned out that was not possible for this particular patient.

You see, he had been taking 8,000 mg of vitamin C per day before going into the hospital for the elective surgery. He hadn't read about all those nasty side effects associated with these huge doses. The dieticians realized there was no way they could replicate that amount of vitamin C using whole foods, so they reluctantly gave him the supplements. That was the only way they could get him healthy again.

It is important to realize that these side effects are rare. One size does not fit all. Just as the beneficial effects of an intervention may not prove beneficial for all concerned, neither will all people experience the side effects. This is similar to prescription pharmaceuticals, which can have numerous side effects listed, yet very few people experience them.

There are a lot of people who take mega doses of vitamin C and claim they haven't been sick since they began that regimen. However, there are also some very well-designed studies conducted by institutions like the Cleveland Clinic that have failed to show any benefit of taking large doses of this vitamin. It does nothing to reduce the instance of infection, nor does it reduce the number of symptom days if a person does get sick.

How can we explain this discrepancy? How can we explain that a well-controlled study done by a highly respected university or a clinical center shows that there is no benefit, yet legions of people find that they stay more healthy when they take this regimen? You cannot dispute data. Numbers are numbers. They are indisputable. However, you always should argue the interpretation of data, and that's what I want to do now.

How do we interpret these valid data coming from the individual experiments with the opposite results being found by the well-controlled studies? First of all, you will always have a potential of a side effect. It doesn't matter what you do. The body does not know the difference between a good effect and a bad effect. As far as the human body is concerned, there is only a biological effect. Whether it is good or bad is an arbitrary determination that we make based upon our desires and our expectations.

Anything that has the potential of having a desirable outcome will always have the potential of having a downside. So, that's really what we're talking about here. Those individuals who experienced a very powerful, positive effect versus those who experienced no effect at all simply are being left vulnerable to the potentially negative side effects. How can we explain it?

Let's return to the ultra-marathoners. A number of studies have been conducted with similar populations, endurance athletes, people who push the envelope. There was one particular study conducted by Dr. Peters, in which a large number of these extreme athletes was recruited, over 70 participants.

They were asked to identify an age-matched control subject; a person who preferably lived in the same environment, perhaps a roommate, who ostensibly would have exposure to the same microbes. This control person could work out, but not run marathons.

The investigators divided each group in half. One half was given 600 mg of vitamin C per day for a period of time corresponding to two weeks until the day of a race. The other half was given a placebo. Nobody knew who was getting what; neither the subjects, nor the people conducting the study. It was a double-blind study.

It was not until the end that the results were revealed, which is the only way you can conduct a study and really trust the interpretation. It was found, among the marathon runners who took that dose of vitamin C, that there was a nearly 50 percent reduction in both the instance of infection as well as the number of symptom days, if indeed, they did get sick. In other words, there's no question that dose of vitamin C did work. It was highly protective in those athletes who took the vitamin C compared with those who took the placebo.

By the way, that was the only dose looked at. We don't know whether more vitamin C would have been more effective, or whether less would have been more effective. Both are possibilities.

Now let's look at the control group, the non-athletes. Vitamin C did nothing. It did nothing to decrease the number of instances of infection, nor did it do anything to reduce the number of infection days.

How do we interpret this? Vitamin C is required only when you need it. You need it if you are increasing your exposure to microbes, and at the same time, putting pressure on those cells whereby they cannot function at a normal level, which is exactly what these athletes are doing.

We talked about catecholamines, epinephrine, and cortisol. What the vitamin C does is to bring those cells back up to normal, back up to where they should be. But in the controls, whose cells are already at normal, there's no added benefit of the vitamin C. And just as well, because you don't ever want more immunity. Too much immunity is what characterizes those people who suffer from an inflammatory-based disease; severe allergies, for example.

Nor, of course, do you want too little immunity. Otherwise, a person might be prone to opportunistic infection. What you always want is an immune system in that healthy mid-range. So, back to that interpretation, why was it that the well-controlled study showed negative effects, while the individuals showed a very positive one? My guess is the well-controlled studies were conducted in those populations that would be least likely to benefit, normal, healthy volunteers.

Stressed out people don't sleep at night, they don't eat healthfully, and they probably aren't going to be bothered to volunteer for any type of clinical study. They'd be rejected anyway, especially if the immune system were an outcome. I've conducted a lot of these types of studies over the years. I don't want stressed out people in any type of experiment where I'm looking at immune outcomes because they'll introduce too much variability.

My guess is the well-controlled studies were conducted in the very population easy to predict would not benefit. In other words, they were the equivalent of the controls in the Peters study. Individuals, however, are not going to care about what happens to the average person in a well-controlled study. All they care about is the fact that they know their lifestyle is giving rise to stressors that are probably unlike anybody else's. If they hear about something that's going to be beneficial, they're going to try it. Those are probably the very people who would be likely to benefit, and the evidence clearly suggests that they do.

Those individuals were volunteering to participate in this uncontrolled experiment. They are using themselves. Some of you may be taking vitamin C yourself. In other words, you are conducting the experiment in your own body. That's exactly what I recommend you do. If something makes sense, give it a try.

However, as you conduct that experiment, do it the way that a scientist would. First of all, make sure there's a need for it. At the same time that you are monitoring the potential beneficial effects of vitamin C, make sure that you are cognizant of the potential downside, and keep track of those symptoms, as well.

Ultimately, what you have to do is decide, do the benefits I derive from taking this drug offset the potential negative, and yes, I am referring to vitamin C as a drug. Operationally, whenever you take anything to bring about a change in your mental or physical well-being, you are defining it as a drug. That means you take the minimum amount required to get the job done. You take it only for the amount of time that you need to have it, and then you stop taking it when the symptoms go away.

Use this process, by the way, for anything that you do to modulate your health. That includes the interventions that might be provided by your pharmacist. The only difference, really, between the drugs that you buy from the health food store and the drugs that you buy from the pharmacist is the FDA requires that in those drugs that have been produced in the laboratory, that certain stringent experiments be conducted to find out what the side effects are so you already know in advance what they are likely to be. We don't know that for the so-called natural products because they are exempt from having to be tested in this manner.

Whether you are experimenting with echinacea, tea tree oil, using mindfulness-based meditation, guided imagery, or behavioral intervention, or whether it's a drug your doctor has prescribed, remember if it has the potential of having a good effect, it will always have the potential of having a downside.

There's another program that I've taught in the past dealing with herbal medicines and alternative medicine. I've lost track of a number of people who would come to those seminars with lists of all of the things that they were taking. They would show it to me and say, "Dr. Hall, is this good for me? Is this helping me stay healthy?"

I would look at them rather puzzled, and say, "Well, that's a question I would ask you. Is it helping you? Why are you taking it?" They're response typically would be, "Well I'm not really sure. I'm just taking it because someone said this would keep me healthy."

It is good to have something you can actually measure and document. If you don't know if something is helping you or not, then don't take the medicine. There's no need for it. You always have to start out with a medical need to intervene. Abide by the rules of taking drugs

One of the things that we all need to remain healthy is sleep. Just about anything that impacts your health is going to directly or indirectly impact the quality of your sleep. I'm going to give you a hypothetical situation and an approach to determining what is beneficial to improving your sleep.

A lot of people wake up and feel exhausted when they get out of bed in the morning despite having slept eight hours uninterrupted. Here's what you want to do. You want to find out if the intervention, whatever it might be, is effective in increasing the amount of energy that you have upon wakening.

Start out by keeping a diary for at least a week, preferably longer. On a scale of one to ten, record how you feel each morning when you first get up. If you feel as though you are in a coma and can barely pick up your crayon to mark the paper, then give yourself a one. If you feel energized, ready to run a marathon, then give yourself a ten.

Do that for a period of at least a week. Then put the notebook away. Don't look at it again. Start a new one after you begin the intervention. Do that for lots of other things too, not just for quality of your sleep: your mood, for example, and the other things that might be important to you.

Then compare the preliminary data you collected, the baseline, with that which you collected after you began the intervention. Remember, the body doesn't know the difference between a good biological effect and a bad one. As far as the body is concerned, a biological effect is a biological effect. Whether it's good or bad is a value judgment that you are making.

At the same time, you are comparing the two diaries, be sure to pay attention, not only to the amount of alertness that you had, but also to the possible downsides. A lot of people decide, "You know what? I wake up with lots more energy, but I feel a little bit more irritable than I used to. I'm not going to worry about it. I like the extra energy; other people are going to have to deal with my irritability." That would be an example of weighing the cost/benefit ratio.

How Your Immune System Works When You're Sick

L et's say we've have gotten to the point where none of this has worked. These secretions have failed to neutralize the microbe at that entry level. The phagocytic cells have been struggling to get rid of the bacteria or virus, but without success, and your immune system is down-regulated because of the large amount of stress and adversity you are facing in your life. You have no choice but to mobilize the A Team. You now need to activate T-cells and the B cells which means more of those pro-inflammatory cytokines in order to mobilize that population of cells. So be prepared to feel lousy.

In microbiology, the symptoms are referred to as sickness behavior. As I mentioned before, inflammation is all about containing the infection. So we now need to bring the lymphocytes close into where the infection is taking place. They enter at the site of injury in much the same way that the phagocytic cells did. However, instead of staying at the site where the viruses happen to be, they are taken up in what are referred to as the lymphatic channels.

The lymphatic channels can be thought of as the biological equivalent of garden hoses which link the various lymph nodes in the body. Lymph nodes are scattered all around. They're found in the groin, the armpits. They line the entire gut. They are also up in your neck area.

It's the lymph node closest to where the infection is taking place which is designated the regional lymph node and that is where all of the action is going to take place. At this stage the different cells have to come together. T-cells, B cells, phagocytic cells, all have to work as a team in order to accomplish the objective of eliminating the virus from the body.

They all come from the same place. That's the pluripotential stem cell found in bone marrow. The T-cells will undergo maturation in the thymus gland. In fact, that's why they are called T-cells. It's because they are thymic dependent. B cells will mature in bone marrow.

Obviously it's not going to do you any good to have that cell sitting up in the thymus gland, or in some distant location in your body when needed in your big toe or down in your lung if you have an upper respiratory infection. So these cells have to get to the area of injury.

They have to migrate out of the thymus gland and travel to where the infection happens to be. We call that lymphocyte trafficking. There are two things that will facilitate trafficking. One is acute stress. Yes, stress affects the release of epinephrine as well as cortisol, such as what we experience all the time with somatic stress, such as exercise.

The hormones at that concentration are not harmful. Indeed, they actually promote your immune system in part by facilitating the migration of the cells from the part of the body where they are maturing to where they are needed. Those cells will migrate through the bloodstream. They'll make their way into the inflamed area, and then they are transported through the lymphatic channels.

The circulatory system has a very powerful pump called the heart. This enables the cells that are within the bloodstream to move very efficiently from one part of the body to another. The lymphatic channels do not have a heart. There is no equivalent pump. What enables the cells to move, albeit very sluggishly, is the peristaltic movement of the muscles surrounding the lymphatic channels.

This is one of the reasons why, if you want to remain healthy, if you want to stay in that preclinical phase, you must exercise. When I discussed the ultra-marathoners and their susceptibility to opportunistic infection, you might have been thinking, "Yes, I'm going to rip up my membership to the gym and donate my running shoes. I knew that exercise was inherently dangerous and now here's the argument to justify quitting."

Not so fast. The ultra-marathoners are about extreme exercise. There is absolutely nothing that will help you to achieve your health goals better than moderate exercise. Indeed, if you want to maintain a state of good health, you must incorporate moderate exercise into your lifestyle.

When you are exercising, you are providing the immune system with the low-to-moderate amounts of cortisol and epinephrine which it needs and at the same time the muscle contractions are facilitating the migration of cells around the body, making sure they are in the right place and at the right time. It's only the extreme exercise that takes a toll on your body, unless of course you take extra protective steps to minimize that possibility.

Once the cells arrive in the lymph node, they are going to undergo cell division. Chemokines are another factor that helps the cells arrive in the right place. We spoke earlier of these chemicals, which help attract the neutrophils and other cells to come in. There are many different types of chemokines, some which bring the T and B cells into the area, which results in in their receiving many other signals in the form of interleukin-1. It used to called T-cell activating factor. That is going to stimulate cell division. Each T and B cell is going to become a daughter cell, which in turn will give rise to two more daughter cells. Each of those will give rise to two more, and so forth.

After a couple of days you will have the equivalent of a flea epidemic taking place on the back of your dog in the middle of August taking place in your lymph node. Except unlike the fleas, which have a carpet to jump onto, they have you to jump onto; the cells have to remain in the confined space of the lymph node, which of course is going to swell up. If it happens to be one of the lymph nodes in your neck, it may be very painful as you turn your neck to look out the side-view window of a car. Rejoice when that happens, provided of course that you have an upper respiratory infection. That is an indication your immune system is doing exactly what it's supposed to be doing.

If you have an upper respiratory infection and your lymph nodes do not swell up, then something is probably wrong. You might be under a lot of duress. You might not be getting healthful sleep. Interleukin-1, which is stimulating the expansion of those cells, is also going to be creating an environment in the body, making it easier for those cells to get the job done.

It turns out that interleukin-1 along with another pro-inflammatory cytokine called interleukin-6 is able to induce a fever response. These two chemical cousins are referred to as pyrogens. Don't run to the medicine cabinet and start popping aspirin every time you run a low-grade fever. A lot of microbes cannot survive when body temperature goes up, even a tiny bit. If they do survive, the entire immune system works more efficiently against a backdrop of elevated temperature.

I live on the Hillsborough River in Tampa, Florida and spend a lot of time on the river in my kayak, and on a cold winter day, it's not uncommon to see a large 12-foot alligator lying on the bank basking in the sun trying to get warmed up. On a cold day, you could actually pull your boat up to the side of the bank, get out, sneak up to that alligator and tap him on the nose.

You'd be really stupid if you were to do that, but you could probably do it and get away with it on a cold winter day because alligators, like all reptiles, are cold-blooded. Their body temperature is the same as the air. So when it cools down, their metabolism slows down as well. They become very sluggish and can barely move.

Don't even think about doing that on a hot summer's day. You'll be lucky if all you lose as your arm. Your lymphocytes are just like that alligator. When they warm up, they become much more agile and more active, and that is why the same IL-1 which is helping to activate these cells is simultaneously acting in the brain along with its cousin IL-6 to make sure there is an environment in the body that is conducive to recovery.

Many cultures have recognized the value of elevated temperature in the healing process, even cultures that knew nothing about the germline theory of disease or anything else about the immune system. Many Native American cultures, for example, prescribed a sweat lodge as a treatment for illness. Their medical paradigm was predicated upon the belief that illness occurred when the body became inhabited by an offended animal spirit.

So the sweat lodge was prescribed as a way of sweating out that spirit. Many of the tribe's prescribed purgatives such as peyote, which would induce vomiting, again for the purpose of expelling that spirit, and even though their interpretation was very different from our interpretation today, the bottom line is the data were correct.

People got better. They got over their symptoms. It worked.

In the Scandinavian countries: Sweden, Norway, Denmark, the sauna is one of the mainstays in medical practice. Of course it came about during a time when disease was thought to be due to evil spirits. But, the intent was exactly the same as that of the Native Americans. Let's flush out these spirits. Get them out of the body. It worked.

Now think about this. What happens when you exercise? You get warm, don't you? You know why? It's because muscles produce a small amount of IL-1 and IL-6. Why should the body have to have separate mechanisms for increasing temperature to accommodate these different systems? How wasteful would that be? So muscles are using exactly the same system.

You're basically running a low-grade fever when you exercise. Imagine early in the morning, somebody's sneezes on you, your little bit groggy, you weren't paying much attention, you didn't take extra precautions, you didn't keep your hands away from your face, so you have that virus incubating in your body. However, you are in the very early phase of a preclinical stage. Everything is getting mobilized.

Later in the afternoon when you go to the gym to work out and you increase your body temperature, chances are that alone will nip it in the bud. You'll provide that extra assist to the innate immune system and you'll never even know how close you came to coming down with clinical symptoms. That is yet another reason why exercise is such a powerful tool to maintain optimal immunity and to stay in that preclinical phase.

The IL-1 along with other cytokines will also help to induce the type of sleep that is extremely beneficial to your immune system. It's referred to as Delta or sometimes as slow-wave sleep. This is the deep, restful stage of sleep which you have to have in order to awaken in the morning feeling fully refreshed, which happens to be when growth hormone is produced.

Growth hormone, as its name implies, stimulates the growth and repair of damaged tissue. Obviously this is something that you would want if a tissue has been damaged by a virus. At the same time it helps to stimulate the growth and expansion of the lymphocytes that you need to move in and help get the job done. It also stimulates the growth and repair of a tissue that's been damaged by the virus.

That is precisely why it is the immune system which facilitates the induction of this particular type of sleep. Yet another benefit of exercise is that it can leave you a little tired shortening the latency of falling asleep and because of that production of IL-1 coming from the muscle, you'll spend more time in Delta sleep.

This would obviously be beneficial to an athlete because that same growth hormone will stimulate the growth and repair of muscle. The same growth hormone is going to be acting on the rest of your body as well, including your immune system.

Wouldn't it be great if you could above and beyond all of this actually manipulate your Delta sleep so you get extra on your terms and exactly when you need it? What if there were a way you could determine when you have first entered the preclinical phase before you have even first symptom that now is the time to take precautions?

There is a way that you can do that. It's very easy. But before I explain it to you, I do need to mention that I am a recovering academic. After spending several decades working in the laboratory researching the links between the brain and the immune system, I became interested in what I refer to as applied psychoneuroimmunology.

Instead of sitting in the lab studying sick people trying to find out what's wrong, trying to gain a better understanding of how and when neurotransmitters and neuropeptides translate an emotion into a signal that impacts the immune system, I became interested in studying very healthy people. What makes them tick? Would there be a way of using that understanding to construct a blueprint that would now help other people to get to that same point?

That meant working with people who were highly successful in athletic endeavors or in corporate America. My first experience in the corporate arena was working with Florida Hospital in Orlando, the nation's largest hospital. At the time they had 14,600 employees and certainly the largest hospital in terms of admission. I worked with them in designing a wellness program for a new community in the Orlando area, which turned out to be hugely successful.

Then the owner of Saddlebrook Resort near Tampa, Florida asked me to establish a similar wellness program that would meet the needs of the professional athletes and corporate clients who gravitate toward that property. Saddlebrook is not the sort of place you would go on vacation. Rather, it is where corporate leaders, Fortune 500 companies, and professional athletes go to attain their next level of performance and to reduce their healthcare costs.

The athletes we work with are people for whom winning is everything, and even the second place silver medal in the Olympics can be regarded as being the first loser. One of my clients was Illbruck Challenge, Germany's entry in the Volvo Ocean Yacht Race, an around the world race, that is very dangerous, and where lives have been lost.

When I asked the team what things they would consider to be a major setback, or the biggest stressor ever experienced, one of the sailors told me it was winning the silver medal in the Olympics. That was one of his greatest disappointments, because he wanted the gold.

So we're talking about extremely high achievers who come to our program. Our reputation would be shot if we made mistakes. At that level of performance, there is really a critical need to exercise daily. For every day that a person takes off, it is likely to take two days to get back to where they were.

That doesn't really apply to weekend warriors like most of us. But when you're at that peak performance level, it's absolutely critical. That means I cannot casually say, "I don't want you to exercise today because I think you're getting sick." If we do say that we'd better be absolutely sure. If we're going to encourage that performer to change his or her training regimen, we'd better be certain that they are about to have some sort of immunological setback.

As I said, for most of us that's irrelevant. For the type of things I do, and probably that you do, we can go the whole week without doing any serious training and then get out there on Saturday afternoon and be as good as you were at the last weekend. But not at the professional level, where the slightest mistake can determine whether or not you're on the podium or you're off to the side.

We've come up with a way to determine when a person is first reaching that preclinical phase, and you can do it too. You'll need to purchase a heart rate monitor. It can be a cheap one. No need to spend more than $50. You don't need to know the barometric pressure. You don't need to know the time in Hong Kong. You certainly don't need a built-in GPS. All you need to know is your heart rate.

Every morning when you get up, sit in your favorite chair, and just totally relax. Don't pick up the morning paper. Don't drink any coffee. Just sit there and relax. You can add Herb Benson's progressive muscle relaxation. You can do some deep breathing or whatever it takes you to get into a state of total relaxation.

It may take several minutes, as you try to see how low your heart rate can go. The lowest is going to be your resting heart rate. Let's say that over a period of several weeks, it's consistently been 60 beats per minute (bpm). Then one morning you get up, and it's 63 bpm.

You stay in the chair a bit longer. You take extra deep breaths. But it's still 63. Obviously you have to be very finely tuned with your body to pick up a change of that small magnitude. The question now is why.

When we're working with the athletes they might report they had an extra glass of wine with dinner at the local restaurant. Okay, no problem. Alcohol dehydrates you, and if you don't compensate by drinking extra water, there will be a very slight decrease in blood volume requiring the heart has to beat a little bit faster to accomplish what it did the day before. No worries. Go out and do whatever the trainers are recommending.

Or, the athlete might tell us, yesterday I took some antihistamines. I have allergies. Okay, no problem. Those dehydrate you too. Go out and do whatever you would normally do.

But, if they can't explain it, if there is absolutely nothing that would explain that increase and especially if there happens to be some bug going around or there are other indications that a person might have been exposed to a virus, then we will surmise that they may very well be in the early stage of a preclinical infection. The immune system is likely producing very small amounts of IL-1 and IL-6, and they may be experiencing a very small increase in body temperature, though not enough to pick up with the drugstore thermometer, but enough to cause a slight dehydration.

When you have an immune response going on, even in the earliest phase, there's going to be increased metabolism. Whenever your metabolism is revved up in any way there's going to be a slight increase in heart rate. We won't tell them not to exercise, in fact will encourage them to work out because we want them to get that body temperature up. We want them to get that extra IL-1 out of their muscles.

But we will also warn them not to push themselves. Just do a light workout, a maintenance workout. Don't push yourself through the zone of discomfort. Not today. Wait.

Then we will have them go to bed 30 minutes earlier than usual. The reason is because throughout the night you cycle through the different stages of sleep. There are four stages that we cycle through. For example, REM sleep (rapid eye movement) is when the brain is in a very active state. If you are awakened from the REM stage you can vividly recall dreams that you were having.

Nobody really knows what the true purpose of sleep is, although there's a lot of evidence to believe that during REM sleep you are rehashing all of the information that came into the brain that day, trying to sort out what to put into long-term storage, what to keep ready at the front burner and so forth. In other words, it is REM sleep that is associated with the consolidation of information into memory.

Non-REM sleep includes Delta or slow-wave sleep, which happens to be a combination of sleep stages three and four. It's the deep, restful sleep I referred to earlier which you must have in order to awaken in the morning feeling refreshed. It's also the stage of sleep where growth hormone is produced which I explained can be very beneficial to the immune system.

If you sleep eight hours, even though you cycle through the stages approximately every 90 minutes, you'll spend proportionately more time in slow-wave sleep during the first half of the cycle. From midnight until 4 AM, for example, and then you spend proportionately more time in REM sleep from four AM till 8 AM. By going to bed 30 minutes earlier than usual, you can actually stack the deck and get extra Delta sleep.

Sleeping in the morning won't do it. That is when you normally get more of the REM. So if you sleep in longer in the morning before getting up, you won't get the neurologic benefits. You won't get that extra Delta. If you do that after determining that your heart rate was up at say 63 bpm and you think you're getting sick, chances are, by going to bed early and awakening the next morning, you'll find that it's back there on to its usual 60 bpm.

I really don't know if that works or not as I cannot do the experiment. I can't walk up to an athlete and say, "I want you to be in this experiment, I think you're about to be sick. There are things I could advise you to do to prevent that. However, I need you to be in the control group." Of course I can't do that. My reputation would be shot. No one would want to come back.

So, what I rely on is the same thing you rely on when you do an experiment to see if something is beneficial. I don't have any data to suggest if this works or not, but what I do have are outcomes. Those outcomes are highly successful athletes. Illbruck Challenge, for example, not only won the Volvo Ocean Race that year. They also set the world record for crossing the Atlantic that year. They were the healthiest and had the fewest instances of infection and were incredibly successful. Therefore I believe it does work. There's no reason you shouldn't try it as well.

Not to mention the benefits of going to bed earlier anyway in order to get that extra energy. You'll know instantly. You'll get immediate gratification that is benefiting you in that regard.

Having this understanding will help you in another way as well. That is, you are going to do just the opposite. If your circumstances only allow you to get a certain amount of very limited sleep each night and you want to make sure when you wake up you are raring to go, then you want to wake up from REM sleep.

That's exactly what happens when you awaken in the middle of the night. You are exhausted when you went to bed only a few hours earlier. You've only slept for an hour and a half but you can't get back to sleep. You're lying there wide-awake and I'm sure that's happened to you.

Wouldn't it be great if you could wake up in the morning during that stage when you need to be getting up? You sleep in 90-minute increments. You cycle through the different stages approximately every 90 to 120 minutes.

That's what I do in the extreme kayak races with Water Tribe. When I pull up to a beach or somebody's dock to catch a few hours of sleep and it's 3 AM, and I know I can only get a few hours of sleep, I'm going to make sure that when I awaken it's at a time when I'm likely to be wide-awake. I don't want to roll over, go back to sleep, and then awaken with the sun beating down and realize that I've missed the tide or there's a storm coming in that now I'm not going to be able to stay ahead of.

What I'll do is time my falling asleep so that my alarm clock goes off at a 90-minute increment at about the same time the sun is coming up. You see, sunlight activates the natural circadian rhythm of cortisol. Cortisol provides you with energy. Remember I spoke about that earlier. Cortisol increases blood glucose and puts pennies into your pocket so you have the energy to do what you need to do.

Levels are highest in the morning. Cortisol is not just produced during stress. It is stimulated by movement and by light when you first get up, providing you with the energy that you need to make it through the day. These are the little tricks that you can do if you work the night shift, if you are traveling, or if there's any reason why you need to be alert when your biological rhythms are telling you that you really ought to be sleeping.

Now a caution, that what I do in those races and what you sometimes have to do, is very unhealthy. There is no question that sleep deprivation, not getting enough sleep, is not only the number one cause of accidents due to human error, especially on the nation's highways, but it is also one of the reasons people suffer miserably from illness.

Sleep deprivation is correlated with heart disease. It's correlated with pro-inflammatory levels of cytokines. So if you suffer any type of inflammation, your symptoms will be very difficult to manage. The really bad thing about it is, if you have been going through a prolonged period of interrupted sleep, it's extremely difficult to get back on track.

Healthy sleep is probably one of the biggest favors you can do, not only for your immune system, but your entire body. Unfortunately, many people regard sleep as the obligatory end of a day. If there is anything you perceive to be pressing, that must be done, it invariably comes out of the sleep column. That is when you do it. You stay up later to finish that task.

If you must finish that report or your tax returns or anything at all, you invariably take the extra time you need away from sleep. Instead of viewing sleep as the obligatory end of a day, I want you to start viewing it as the essential beginning of the next day.

Everything is going to be contingent on getting helpful sleep, including your mood, your immune system, and all you need to have in place to achieve your objectives and success that day The average person needs between seven and ten hours. Exactly where you fall varies from individual to individual.

The basic rule of thumb is you need enough. If you have to awaken to an alarm clock, you're probably not getting enough. It's that simple. By the way the information that I'm giving you is probably going to wipe out the one excuse that you use to not exercise. That is, I don't have time.

One of the benefits of exercise is not just for your immune system, but for the quality of your sleep. Exercise actually enables you to generate time. You will manufacture minutes. The reason is because of IL-1 and getting that extra Delta sleep. As a consequence, you'll spend more time in deep, restful sleep, enabling you to sleep more efficiently and probably awaken before the alarm clock goes off.

Once people start doing this, they report waking 10 to 15 minutes before the alarm clock. You multiply that extra ten minutes per day by seven days a week by 365 days a year and you're going to generate the time that you spent exercising because you don't have to do that much in order to maintain optimal immunity.

Most studies show working out a minimum of three days a week for 30 minutes at a time, not even running, just brisk walking, is really all you need to do. Obviously, if you want to build up cardiovascular fitness, you need to be in the aerobics zone, or if you are training for a master sporting event, you need to do it for longer. But for the immune system, it doesn't take that much.

Let's factor in because you woke up so refreshed, you can do things more efficiently during the day. As a result, you'll pick up extra time as a result of that. You may even end up with surplus time, not just the time you spent exercising. And it's your time.

You can do whatever you want with it. You can add it to the pleasure column or the productivity column. You can even spend more time exercising and reap greater benefits. So you can no longer use the excuse "I don't have time." "I don't feel like it" or "I don't look good in spandex" are still available excuses. However, you cannot use "I don't have time." Not anymore.

I want you to think for just a minute how you felt the last time you were really sick, as in flat on your back. Achy, fever, fatigue, lethargy, and what happened to your appetite? What appetite? Were you motivated to go out and do anything? Of course not. These are the symptoms of depression.

There's a manual used by psychologists to diagnose mental illness. It's called the DSM-V and you will find just about every one of these symptoms in the chapter called Depression. You'll also find them in virtually any immunology textbook, but you won't find the word depression. You'll find those symptoms described in the section of the book with the title Sickness Behavior. In the context of having an infection every one of these symptoms is extremely beneficial. They are so beneficial that I will dare say that if you are a parent, at one time or another you have encouraged your child to act depressed.

I've done that. Stay in bed today. Don't worry about going to school. Don't go to the concert. Don't worry about eating. Just drink lots of fluid. This is something my wife and I have been telling our children the whole time they were growing up, because we recognized the benefits. It is so beneficial going into behavioral withdrawal that it's actually coordinated by the immune system.

The symptoms of depression you experience when you are sick are actually induced by pro-inflammatory cytokines. Before I explain which ones are doing what,

I'll quickly point out that what we are really dealing with here is a shift in motivation. The shift from a desire to engage in behaviors that would normally give rise to pleasure, that will now give rise to optimal immunity and speed our recovery from illness.

We don't call it depression in microbiology circles. We call it merely a shift in motivation to quickly recover and for reasons that I'm about to explain. You don't want to be out there exposing yourself to other microbes when you are fighting the one that you've already got. This is because your immune system becomes down-regulated while you are fighting a particular infection.

Here's why. When most lymphocytes are expanding it is only going to be the cells that you need for that particular attack. If you've been exposed to influenza A, then it's only the T-cells and B-cells that respond to influenza A that will be undergoing cell division. The rest of the cells are just standing by waiting, just in case you get a streptococcus infection or anything else.

The ones with specificity for other things are not affected. Part of the signal that turns on the necessary T-cells will be dendritic cells which represent a fragment of the infecting bacteria or virus which ensures you get the right population of cells turned on. This is all going on back in the lymph node. This takes an enormous amount of energy.

You think your fuel bill was high last winter? You should see what the immune system has to pay to run even a low-grade fever. It's astronomical. It's obscene. To facilitate cell division, production of cytokines, antibody production, you need a lot of energy. So where does the energy come from? It comes from cortisol. IL-1 will actually stimulate cortisol release by acting in the brain.

The same steroid that mobilizes energy for the fight/flight response when you are running away from a predator or fighting something in the external environment is exactly the same system which is mobilized when you are fighting a virus or bacteria. Why wouldn't it be? Why waste a perfectly good system for mobilizing energy sources in vastly different ways. Let's be efficient about this.

You have all of these wonderful things going on, the increase in temperature, the growth hormones that are facilitating an increase in immunity, so why on earth would you have production of cortisol, which has the potential of down regulating the whole system? It turns out it's not a problem. As the cells undergo maturation, the ones in the lymph nodes that are fighting that influenza lose their steroid receptors.

The ones that you need right now to fight off that virus escape the potential inhibitory influence of cortisol, which happens to be going up. But the cells that haven't been activated, the ones that are standing by, have not lost their receptors. So they are going to be vulnerable to the infection. The cells that are standing by are going to be vulnerable to the effects of cortisol. It's called antigenic competition.

An antigen is anything that stimulates the immune system. While the immune system is fighting one antigen, your ability to fight off others is going to be impaired. That is exactly why the immune system makes sure you stay in bed. Stay out of the village. You don't want to be exposing yourself to other things when you are more vulnerable.

It's not at all uncommon for people to come down with an immobilizing streptococcus infection when they have the flu. Streptococcus is a bacteria. The flu is a virus. Virtually any virus, while you're fighting it, is going to have this small amount of immunosuppressive activity.

It would be nice to think that there's an altruistic imperative here as well. That perhaps the human body has come up with a system so you don't go out and infect other members of the community. I doubt seriously that is part of the biological imperative, but it would be nice to suppose it is.

That is one of the reasons why it is important to space out vaccines if possible. I know that when the H1N1 influenza was a threat to people living in this country at the same time seasonal flu was, the Florida Department of Public Health recommended that people space out the timing of these two vaccines. Allow two weeks between them in order to avoid this antigenic competition in order to get the maximum amount of protection.

I know that a lot of people are concerned about the practice of giving multiple vaccines to very young children. There are different arguments, pros, and cons in favor of this protocol. One is being offered by the Public Health Service which is responsible for the overall health of the population. The other would be the recommendations being made by individual health professionals, physicians, for example, who are responsible for their patients' individual health.

From a population standpoint, you want to vaccinate as many people as you can with whatever you can get into them at the opportunity. If a single mom who is struggling to make ends meet, who can barely afford to get her kids into the doctor's office and can only get there one time, then go ahead give that child as many vaccines as possible while that child is there because some protection is better than none. From a public health standpoint, that is a very wise decision.

But, if you can afford it, and the doctor will work with you spacing out the vaccine so you can avoid this antigenic competition, then that is probably the way to go. You'll optimize the response against each one. There are always exceptions. DPT is a triple vaccine. It turns out that the pertussis, which is protective against whooping cough, serves to adjuvant, or augment, the antibody titer against the diphtheria and the tetanus.

That is the exception. Adjuvants often added to vaccines in order to provide this priming. Adjuvants will nonspecifically mobilize the immune system. But in this particular vaccine, not only is one of the antigens (P) itself eliciting the production of memory cells to protect the person from pertussis later on, it is also augmenting response to the D and the T, the diphtheria and the tetanus.

To make sure it is operating optimally, your immune system provides signals to the brain to create infection fighting behaviors. How does this happen? In one example, Interferon alpha acts to speed up the recycling of serotonin in the brain.

It's basically doing the opposite of selective serotonin reuptake inhibitors, drugs like Zoloft and Prozac. It'll speed up the recycling; thereby limiting the time the serotonin would normally be available, and I think you probably know that that correlates with some forms of clinical depression.

Some of the pro-inflammatory cytokines are able to redirect the conversion of tryptophan from serotonin to a pathway that gives rise to kynurenic acid. It is impairing as well the conversion of serotonin into leucine-1. Leucine-1 is capable of binding to GABA receptor, gamma aminobutyric acid receptors, in the brain. That's what Valium binds to. No wonder you feel emotionally flat when you are sick.

Interferon binds to opioid receptors. That was one of my contributions in the field. Beta-endorphin which binds to opioid receptors is the body's endogenous morphine. That's what the word means. So when you bind to receptor with interferon alpha you're going to prevent the body's natural pain killer endorphin from attaching. That's what the word means. It's like putting chewing gum into the lock preventing the key from getting in. No wonder you feel lousy. All of these things collectively are making sure you have no motivation to do what you would normally do and that you will engage in behaviors that are going to be conducive to conserving energy to make it available to the immune system. In other words, depression is prewired. Problems arise when you continue to suffer and you have no energy, because now these pro-inflammatory cytokines are continuing to be produced in excess.

I would now like to introduce you to another type of individual. A woman most likely in her late 20s or early 30s, bright, athletic, works out on a regular basis. Extremely healthy, rarely get sick, gets up feeling fully refreshed each morning, puts on her $800 Ann Klein suit, prepares a nutritious breakfast for her 2.6 children which they eat, drops her children off at school, and then goes off to her own socially meaningful and worthwhile job where she earns a six-figure salary.

She runs several miles on her lunch break, and then goes home at the end of the day to prepare a gourmet meal for her family, discusses the economic trends with her husband, and then goes to bed, has multiple orgasms, falls into a deep, restful sleep, awakens a few minutes before the alarm clock the next morning ready to start the day afresh.

What I have just described is superwoman as penned by the columnist Ellen Goodman. But Ellen Goodman might just as well have described the perfect candidate for chronic fatigue syndrome, a young healthy woman, who rarely gets sick, who is successfully balancing work and family, who comes down with a rare infection. It's very unusual for her, but eventually when she recovers the virus has been put into remission. Her immune system continues to produce those pro-inflammatory cytokines, the ones capable of acting in the brain. They keep going on and on. Just like the Energizer Bunny, inducing lethargy. This is basically one explanation for that elusive condition referred to as chronic fatigue syndrome.

We're talking about chronic fatigue syndrome, which is not a real disease. It's exactly what its name says it is. It's a syndrome. By definition, a syndrome is a collection of many symptoms. There may be many circumstances that give rise to the same symptoms. Now the symptoms are very real. There is very good evidence to believe that some forms of chronic fatigue syndrome may be due to a runaway immune system, in other words, excessive production of these pro-inflammatory cytokines.

Why did they run out of control? Because of a normal braking system that keeps the immune system in the help a mid-range is no longer functioning. That braking system happens to be cortisol. No, cortisol did not evolve for the purpose of rendering you sick. Cortisol is the body's natural means by which to keep the immune system in that healthy mid-range, to keep it from going up too high.

Research with a strain of rat, the Lewis rat, in the laboratory of Esther Sternberg at the National Institutes of Health, suggests that when cortisol production is low, when it drops down below a critical threshold, it results in a chemical cascade, resulting in overproduction of immune cytokines.

In the model that Doctor Sternberg uses, it's due to the absence of corticotropin-releasing hormone, the chemical in the brain that ultimately gives rise to elevated cortisol. As a result of lacking this potentially immunosuppressive hormone, the rats' immune systems are such that when they are exposed to basic myelin protein, they develop the symptoms of multiple sclerosis, an autoimmune disease characterized by too much immunity attacking basic myelin protein.

In other words, the immune system keeps attacking the myelin sheath because there is no steroid to bring it back down. This is a hypothesis. It has not been proven and certainly not in humans. And it does not apply to all states of chronic fatigue syndrome. However, it may explain some circumstances of this debilitating condition.

How Your
Mind Affects Your
Immune System

'm going to switch gears and emphasize the brain, but not in the way that cytokines are acting upon the nervous system. We are going to focus on the way your thoughts, your emotions are capable of influencing the ability of white cells to fight viruses. The mind is capable of influencing the immune system in many ways.

That includes the characteristics that comprise what we refer to as personality. During the 1960s, psychiatrist Doctor George Solomon, one of the pioneers in the field of psychoneuroimmunology, conducted a very interesting study. He observed among identical twins that one would develop rheumatoid arthritis, whereas the other would not.

He was curious about this. After all, they were identical. They had the exact same immune response genes. They grew up in identical environments. They ate from the same supply of food, drank from the same supply of water. Indeed, they had the same parental upbringing.

It turned out that the distinguishing feature of the person who developed the arthritis is what he referred to as the rheumatoid arthritic personality: a person who is very accommodating, someone who will put their own emotional needs on a back burner to care for the needs of others, person who essentially says, "Yes" when they want to say, "No." They are also people who have a very difficult time dealing with anger, expressing it in themselves as well as in other people. The first time that another person is about to get angry, they will do whatever they need to do to keep that person on an even keel.

Dr. Lydia Temoshok had just received her PhD in clinical psychology at Yale University and was very interested in this work. She began a postdoctoral fellowship with Dr. Solomon, further characterizing this correlation between the rheumatoid arthritic individual and the one who was free of those symptoms and then wrote the bestselling book *The Type C or Cancer Connection.*

She discovered that not only are these individuals prone to inflammatory based disease, but they are also more likely to develop cancer, especially malignant melanoma. I'm not talking about the kind of malignant melanoma that occurs when you spend too much time basking in the sun or utilizing tanning beds.

I'm referring to the type of person who is darker complexioned whose melanoma shows up on the inside of their gum, the sole of their foot, their armpit, places that seldom see intense sunlight. When those individuals develop melanoma, invariably they have the type C personality. The type C individual has also been found to have elevated levels of interleukin-6. Interleukin-6, if you will recall, is one of the pro-inflammatory cytokines and that is exactly what you would predict in a person who is going to be prone to inflammatory based disease, such as rheumatoid arthritis.

Dr. Temoshok went on to work in the laboratory of Dr. Robert Gallo, the co-discoverer of HIV. He was running one of the most powerful immunology labs in the country. Normally a virologist such as Dr. Gallo would no sooner talk to a behaviorist than he would share the same toothbrush.

So what is a clinical psychologist doing in one of the most successful virology labs in the country? They have discovered that the type C individual is more likely after exposure to HIV to progress to full-blown AIDS much more rapidly than the non-type C. It appears to be related to their CD4-positive lymphocytes, the T helper population which is largely responsible for coordinating the efforts of all of the other immune system cells.

What Dr. Temoshok discovered is that these CD4-positive cells have an altered chemokine receptor. Remember, that's the receptor, which responds to the chemical magnet drawing the cells to where they are needed. There are very pronounced and important biochemical changes that exist in these people that basically communicate that they have a dis-regulated immune system.

The question now is how do you measure the type C individual? How do you determine that it exists? One of the characteristics of these people is they have a very high need for social desirability. They need to be liked. Not only that, they will rarely admit to even expressing the emotion of anger.

If you ask a person who is a type C, "When was the last time you were angry?" They'll spend a lot of time thinking about it. "Well, I'm sure that I've been angry once because everybody gets angry. Don't they? Let me see if I can think of when that was." If you asked that same question of a type A, they'll be more likely to respond by saying, "Well I'm angry right now. You kept me waiting for this appointment." They'll be able to tell you half a dozen when they were angry and just in the last couple of hours.

The type A individual is basically the opposite of the type C. They are people who are time oriented, always looking at their watches, never taking time out to smell the roses. They often speak with a very rapid rate of speech finishing your sentences for you because they get impatient waiting for you to finish saying whatever it is you're going to say, probably because whatever you have to say is not worth listening to in the first place.

It's a person who is basically in a win-lose mode: "I'm going to win. You're going to lose. We are going to do it my way or not at all." Whereas the type C is in the lose-win mode: "I'm going to lose. You're going to win. Your needs are far more important than mine." It's very interesting that whereas the type C individual is more prone to inflammatory disease, the type A's are far more likely to have a heart attack or succumb to a stroke.

You might think that there's somewhat of a contradiction here. After all, inflammation is associated with too much immunity: excessive production of proinflammatory cytokines. However, defense against cancer requires natural killer cells: cytotoxic T-cells. In other words, it would seem then that a person who has a revved up immune system who also happens to have cancer would actually benefit from that enhanced immunity that increased inflammation.

So how can it be that we have the same personality prone to inflammatory disease, which is too much immunity and cancer which is thought to be associated with too little? There really is no contradiction. That's because inflammation plays a critical role in the growth and metastases of cancer, which refers to the spread of cancer from its origin to other locations in the body.

There are two ways this can happen. One is through intrinsic inflammation, whereby the cancer cell itself produces the pro-inflammatory cytokines. The other is extrinsic, whereby the cancer will take over a nearby inflammatory process but utilize it in a way that promotes its own growth and expansion.

In intrinsic inflammation results in activation of oncogenes, such that the cancer cell will start producing much of the same substances I spoke about previously. However, instead of turning on other lymphocytes, instead of promoting the growth of other cells that are needed in inflammation, they will promote the growth of the cancer.

Probably one of the most dangerous cells recruited into the area is what is referred to as the tumor-associated macrophage. It starts producing large amounts of enzymes. However, instead of chewing up bacteria and viruses, it starts to release these enzymes to break down the matrix of tissue surrounding the tumor, allowing it to escape and move out into the rest of the body.

Cytokines are produced, as are chemokines, those chemical messengers which attract cells into the nearest lymph node. The cancer is turning this all around, so that the chemokine being produced serves as a chemical magnet pulling the cancer to the nearest lymph node and, of course, from there it can spread even further. At the same time, it's capable of activating a type of regulatory T-cell called the suppressor cell. This effectively turns off those elements of the immune system which might otherwise be capable of fighting the cancer.

In the gap, it's more likely that the cancer is going to be using extrinsic information if a person has H. pylori infection, a punitive trigger of ulcers. If they have colitis or for that matter any type inflammation going on within the digestive area, a cancer that develops in that region is likely to basically reach out and grab onto the inflammatory products and then promote its own growth in much the same way I described for the others.

So far the trials indicate that it is sometimes more effective to treat a person. Currently there are clinical trials underway pairing anti-inflammatory drugs with traditional chemotherapeutic agents. The evidence so far suggests that combining the chemotherapeutic drug with an anti-inflammatory is more effective than pairing the chemotherapy with a placebo. It's going to be a long time before this approach ever makes it to a point where it can be safely used as an intervention. The reason is a lot of cancers are eliminated because of inflammation. You need the inflammation to help get rid of the tumor especially when it involved mobilization of natural killer cells.

Decades ago a German physician discovered an endotoxin which when injected into his patients caused the cancer to seemingly disappear. No large-scale clinical trial was ever undertaken. It was mostly anecdotal evidence. The first trials were planned at one point to be carried out in the United States. They were referred as the coli endotoxins. That was before efficient transportation was available and so the culture of bacteria that was being used to generate this toxin was lost as it was being transported across the Atlantic Ocean, but there is now renewed interest in using these endotoxins.

It appears that they may be serving as an adjunct, which helps to non-specifically mobilize both components of the immune system, which may now be able to benefit the patient who suffers from this chronic disease, so there's no contradiction. Whatever it is about the type C individual that makes them prone to inflammation is also going to be an advantage for certain types of cancers for individuals who have that particular genetic blueprint. But now that I have told you that there are these different personalities, I'm now going to tell you that they really don't exist. There's no such thing as a type A or type C personality.

We are all composites of all of these personalities. In fact, I hope you are. I hope you have what is used to be called 'multiple personality disorder.' I hope you don't interact with your children in the way you interact with your colleagues. I hope you're not the same person as you sit here reading that you would be if you were at New Year's Eve party or if you're just been cut off on the interstate highway. I hope that what we call personality does change, so it's now appropriate for the circumstances.

The fact is what we call a personality is really a coping style. It's the way we cope, the way we respond to the environment. The reason I don't like that word *personality* is that it implies permanence. There is nothing wrong with any of these personalities. There's nothing wrong with being a type C. Thank goodness that every one of our mothers was a hardcore card-carrying professional type C when we were infants and our survival depended upon her nurturing, when it depended upon her sacrificing her need for sleep and lots of other things in order to care for us.

But it's not okay for Mom to be a type C when she's the patient in the hospital, then waits until her throat is parched before troubling the staff for a glass of water and only to apologize for having taken the staff's time. That is a very unhealthy style to have in that particular environment.

And there is nothing wrong with being a type A. Sometimes there is justification to express anger, to be impatient. It was Aristotle who argued that to withhold anger when it is justified was a vice, not a virtue, that anger basically motivates other people to change their behavior, to alert them that they have wronged you.

There's nothing wrong with any emotion including those associated with the type A; and if something needs to be done very quickly, if people who are not getting the job done need to be kicked out of the way, so that progress can be made, then that's the role of the type A.

These are coping styles. The truly healthy individual, the person who is going to achieve a state of optimum health is a person who will be a composite of all of these. It's a person who is assertive or aggressive when they need to be. It's a person who is compassionate and altruistic when that is called for; and that is what we refer to as the type B individual, truly a composite of the two.

Let's consider what would happen if you are a type C. If you are an individual who for whatever reason is susceptible to inflammation, and please remember we are only dealing with a correlation. There is certainly reason to believe that the personality comes first and then as a result of the coping strategy, this now leads to changes in the immune system. The evidence is that these folks often were abused as children by adults. They learned at a very early age that in order to stay safe, they would need to make sure that the adult in their life did not become angry and the first hint that the person was about to get upset, they would step in and do whatever they could to keep that person calm, to keep from being hit. That is what they learned as a child and it carried out into adulthood as the strategy they continued to use.

On the other hand, given what I've been speaking about regarding the ability of cytokines to act in the brain and affect things that are oftentimes related to your personality, one could argue that perhaps it's the immune system that is bringing about this coping style. For years some of the greatest minds studying emotions, people like Claude Bernard, Walter Cannon, argued are you running away because you are afraid, or are you afraid because you are running away. You obviously can't be afraid, you can't be angry. You can't be in love unless there's a trigger. There has to be an object of that emotion. However once the emotion is set in place, there are chemical changes that occur throughout the body and those chemicals in many cases are capable of feeding back to the brain to potentiate the emotion.

As those great minds were doing their research in the early part of the last century, they realized that in fact emotions come from every cell in the body and so it may be true of the immune system and type C coping style. There obviously has to be some sort of event that triggers the original change. However as a result of pro-inflammatory cytokines being produced in excess, perhaps somehow they react in the brain to potentiate that coping style, that personality if you prefer to call it that.

We must realize that right now we don't really know for sure which one is the horse and which is the cart. Whenever you have any type of correlation, you always to consider reverse causality, so at this point all we have is a correlation.

What Can We Do About Inflammation?

Are there things that you can do in order to negate some of the symptoms of inflammation? There certainly are. Let's begin with what it is that people are really concerned about and that's the pain and discomfort. This is due to prostaglandins. Prostaglandins are a crucial part of the overall inflammatory response and they work in concert with leukotrienes, which are largely responsible for bringing cells into the area and both the leukotrienes and the prostaglandins come from a fatty acid called arachidonic acid. If you could somehow control the amount of arachidonic acid and its ability to be converted to prostaglandins, that clearly would be a strategy to better manage the pain and discomfort associated with inflammation.

Hold that thought for a just a moment and what I would like to do now is have you project your mind in space and time to the 1950s. Mr. Ray Kroc founded McDonald's and all of the other fast food chains jumped on the bandwagon. In the 1960s approximately half of the American diet was comprised of fat. Then it was recognized that there seemed to be an association with that and people having their first heart attack in their early 40s. As often happens, we overreacted and started demonizing fat and that's when foods were being sold with fat-free or reduced-fat labels on them.

But then lipid biochemists came along and said you know it's not really all fats that are bad. It's the saturated fats, which tend to clog up the arteries. The unsaturated fats are okay. And then further research was done and it was decided that not all polyunsaturated fats were beneficial. The Omega-3 fatty acids are good, but the Omega-6s were declared bad. Why would they say that?

Omega-6 fatty acids speed up the formation of prostaglandins, in other words they are pro-inflammatory. However the Omega-3 fatty acids do just the opposite. They are anti-inflammatory. The fact is you need both of them. You need both of them to stabilize cell membranes. They are referred to as essential fatty acids, which means you have to get them from the diet. You can't make them yourself.

Remember, you need inflammation. Inflammation is how we get rid of viruses, bacteria, but we don't need the excessive amount of Omega-6s that comprise the average American diet. If you want to undertake a strategy to control inflammation, then reduce the amount of arachidonic acid that is available. Once the arachidonic acid is present take steps to reduce its conversion into prostaglandins and leukotrienes. If you want to take control of inflammation you can eliminate those dietary ingredients that are likely to give rise to inflammation.

It's a no-brainer to cut out those foods that are rich in arachidonic acid. Fish have a very low arachidonic acid index, while certain meats, especially organ meats are very, very high. The Atlantic herring for example has an arachidonic index of one. Many fish are in the single digits as well. If you want to take in extra arachidonic acid, then eat foods such as beef liver, a good steak and kidney pie. There are some cultures such as mine that would consider these as comfort foods, but if you suffer from inflammation, these are not foods that you really want to be ingesting, if you want to control the pain and discomfort.

My recommendation is this. If you suffer from inflammation or at times when you are likely to have a flare-up, examine all the foods that you enjoy, and then select those that are lower on the arachidonic acid index and avoid those that are higher. Do the same for the glycemic index. The glycemic index is a measure of how rapidly a food is converted into blood sugar. Carbohydrates tend to be much higher than other macro nutrients, and among the carbohydrates some are very, very high, such as refine white bread. The faster your blood sugar goes up, the more insulin your pancreas will produce, and insulin does just the opposite of what cortisol does.

Remember we're talking about an energy transaction. Cortisol is writing the withdrawal slip in the body's biological banks. When you need energy, it's pulling it out of storage making it available. Insulin is writing the deposit slip, so any extra sugar that you have is put into storage by the insulin. It turns out that when you eat a large amount of refined sugar or foods that are quickly converted into sugar, the insulin will go up very rapidly and that insulin will speed up the formation of arachidonic acid. That's why people who develop anti-inflammatory diets will include foods that are low in their ability to be converted into sugar, and completely eliminate refined sugar. That means no sweetened soda.

A lot of these drinks dispensed by vending machines are nothing more than liquid sugar with some caffeine and flavoring added. Many people experience almost instantaneous relief simply by cutting back on Coke and other soft drinks.

There are other things you can do as well. For example there are drugs available that will slow down the conversion of arachidonic acid into prostaglandins. The enzyme responsible for doing this is called cyclooxygenase. Many of the anti-inflammatory drugs available are cyclooxygenase inhibitors, such as Celebrex, aspirin or ibuprofen.

I'm not opposed to using DuPont's recommendation, which was "better living through chemistry." I am emphasizing behavioral interventions and the things that you can do in more of a natural realm, because these things don't cost you any money. At the same time an enormous amount of research has been done to improve the quality of people's lives through pharmacology. You'd be crazy not to take advantage of this research, especially if pain and discomfort are interfering with your quality of life. However, some people are concerned about the potential side effects and rightfully so.

My recommendation is to combine it all by eating those foods that tend to be lower on the arachidonic acid index along with those foods that tend to be lower in the ability to be converted into sugar. While you're certainly not going to wipe out all the symptoms completely, you're not going to make the disease disappear; you will at least make the symptoms a little more manageable, so the drug you take will be just as effective at a lower concentration, thereby reducing the likelihood of side effects. Perhaps the pain will subside enough that you can go out and exercise, which will trigger for a release of beta endorphin that will help mask pain. Remember endorphin means endogenous morphine.

At the same time the movement, the exercise, will result in elevated cortisol. That's because of the demands you are putting on your body, so cortisol is probably going to be the chemical released to provide increased sugar in your bloodstream. But recall that cortisol is also the body's most powerful anti-inflammatory hormone. Before you know it, the symptoms won't be there at all. The disease is still there. It's simply reaches the point where the symptoms are not interfering with your productivity or your capacity for pleasure. Combining these types of interventions will enable you to make the difference. You will find that you can control the most important part of the process and that is what gives rise to the symptoms.

By the way I realize that eating is one of the few pleasures we get to enjoy that is still legal, so I strongly recommend that you do not allow the science of nutrition to interfere with the art of eating. I'm not suggesting you eat foods that are not palatable to you just to accomplish some biological objective. Be sensible about it. I'm suggesting is to look at all the foods you enjoy, and favor those that are likely to give you some relief at times when you have inflammation. And if inflammation is not a problem for you, then go ahead and make these recommendations to others, but don't worry about it yourself.

I spoke earlier about the ability of some of these pro-inflammatory cytokines that you are now trying to control to impact the brain. Specifically I emphasized those which were capable of inducing depression. One could argue that if there are certain foods capable of attenuating inflammation, there might be some combination of foods that would be effective as anti-depressants.

Interestingly there's been an article in the archives of *General Psychiatry* reporting exactly that. It was a survey done with over 10,000 people in Spain examining the impact of the Mediterranean diet upon depression. It turns out that those individuals who adhered to the basically anti-inflammatory Mediterranean diet were significantly less likely to become clinically depressed, which is exactly what you would predict given the role the current inflammatory cytokines play in triggering some forms of depression.

The Mediterranean diet is a very sensible diet. You're not restricting yourself of anything at all. There is meat in that diet, but not very much. Most of the animal protein is derived from fish, which is also a source of the anti-inflammatory Omega-3 fatty acid. Not only that, there is a large amount of monounsaturated fatty acids that are associated with the olive oil they consume. These monounsaturated fatty acids seem to be able to cause serotonin to bind more strongly to receptors. Remember elevated serotonin is what you want when you are depressed.

There's a lot of carbohydrate in this diet especially in the form of whole grain breads and cereals. Another ingredient is a moderate amount of especially red wine, not a small amount, but moderate consumption of red wine, which contains flavonoids and resveratrol and other benefits. These are just some of the things that you can do. The key to all of this is moderation.

One of the questions that I've often been asked because my research delved into this is how do these cytokines get into the brain? After all the brain is protected by a blood-brain barrier, which keeps large proteins such as the cytokines out, so how do they exert these effects on body temperature, on depression, on sleep? When I was activity doing research in this area, somebody in the audience after I presented the data would raise their hand and say, "Nick, this is very interesting study, very elegant experiments, but you're a scientist. How do you explain how these substances get across into the brain?"

And I would respond by saying you're absolutely right. As you know there really isn't much of a blood-brain barrier around the ventricles, the area postrema, and other locations. Also there is evidence that when blood pressure goes up, the blood-brain barrier becomes a little leaky, and that is how these things get in. And the person who'd asked the question would nod in agreement and say, "Yes, I accept that answer."

Well, I didn't and neither did the handful of other people who were working in this esoteric area in the early 1980s when we were trying to first explore whether or not there was a connection between the brain and the immune system. I knew the areas where the compounds were being affected were protected by a blood-brain barrier and that was the perplexing question, how do they get in?

A few years ago it was discovered that they don't need to get in. Here is an analogy with the perception of pain. When you place your hand on a hot stove, the sensation of heat is not transmitted to your brain. If it were, the spinal cord would be cooked. No, the intense heat stimulates pain receptors along with temperature receptors. Then the signal is transduced into an electrical message, which shoots up the spinal cord spinning off a reflex along the way, so you can move your hand before the pain is even perceived; and then a millisecond or two before it arrives in the brain, it's interpreted as a signal, which is translated into extreme pain associated with heat. That is how the cytokines work.

If you have inflammation going on in the gut associated with food poisoning, food allergy or perhaps H.
pylori in the stomach, the cytokines being produced
will stimulate the ends of the nerves that are part of the
vagal afferent branch, which some people regard as a
third branch of the autonomic nervous system. Unlike
the other two branches of the autonomic nervous system,
the sympathetic and parasympathetic, which transmit
messages from the brain down to the rest of the body,
the vagal afferent branch transmit messages from the
internal organs back up to the brain.

When interferon alpha is being produced in the gut,
it will send its own unique electrical signature up the
nerve, which is interpreted by neurons on the brain as
meaning we need to produce interferon alpha up here in
the central nervous system. The message is transferred
over to another cell, a microglia cell, which happens to be
the brain's macrophage, which then cranks up production
of that cytokine or interleukin-1 or interleukin-6 and so
on. So these chemical messages don't have to get into
the brain. They might, but they don't need to because
they can signal their production within neurons through
these pathways.

Probably one of the most common sources of inflammation that at lot of people totally ignore is gum disease. The reason many people ignore is because often
the pain is relatively mild. You can avoid it by simply
chewing food on the other side. The only evidence that
something might be amiss is the drop of blood in your

toothpaste when you brush your teeth. I can assure you that if the gums are inflamed enough that they are resulting in production of chemicals that cause discomfort or most certainly if they are damaged sufficiently by this inflammatory process that blood is now leaking out into saliva, you surely have production of pro-inflammatory cytokines, which will now stimulate the ends of the glossopharyngeal nerve which innovates the upper palate.

That electrical signal is conveyed through those nerves into the brain. If you are suffering from lethargy, fatigue, or have no motivation, you know what to do, but you just won't do it, or any other related symptom that is associated with what I've been speaking about make certain you get your thyroid checked out. Make sure you don't have a metabolic disorder, but at the same time you're trying to get a handle on what's going on, visit your dental hygienist. Pay a visit to your dentist because the problem may very well reside in your mouth. In fact that may be the sole cause of your problem.

By the way, if the gums are inflamed sufficiently that blood is leaking out of the circulation and getting into salvia, then obviously the bacteria giving rise to the plaque, resulting in the inflamed gums can get into the bloodstream. And where do you suppose it might end up? The heart. There is indeed a very strong correlation between inflammation and heart disease, so if patients have other risk factors for heart disease; the doctor will routinely call for a measure of their C reactive protein as part of their annual physical. This is an acute phase protein that doesn't tell you where the inflammation is located or caused by. All it tells you is that somewhere in the body inflammation is going on. Oftentimes that information will be associated with the heart, which is why many doctors will look at elevated C reactive protein levels with a great deal of concern, especially if their heart patient is a smoker lives a sedentary lifestyle and is obese.

There's something else that inflammation is associated with. Do you know that most suicides occur in the spring and fall? The reason is not because of daylight savings time. It's not because of the correlation with certain major family events and so forth. It's because those are the allergy seasons in the United States. Spring is the main allergy season triggered by tree pollen. Fall is the secondary season most likely triggered by ragweed, although of course there lots of other things that people might be allergic to and not necessarily just during those timeframes, but those are the peak seasons.

That runny nose, the teary eyes and all of the stuffiness you experience is what we call rhinitis, which is inflammation of the nasal passages. You're producing the same pro-inflammatory cytokines, which tickle the end of the olfactory nerve. That's the conduit used to transmit messages up into the brain. Now, we know that neither these pro-inflammatory cytokines nor allergies cause suicide, but in a person who is on the edge, who is despondent, who has other risk factors and now has allergy, triggering the cytokines may become the proverbial straw that breaks the camel's back.

In the last half dozen years we've come to realize that inflammation in many ways is the Holy Grail of medicine and certainly of psychoneuroimmunology. Inflammation or by extension the immune system is doing a lot more than simply fighting off bacteria and viruses, and in some cases helping to protect us against cancer. It's involved in things we never even dreamed it would be involved in. Psychoneuroimmunology, neuroimmunomodulation, psycho-neuroendocrine-immunology, these are the words that I use to describe this field. Other expressions: the mind/body connection, mind over matter. Every one of these words, every one of these expressions denotes the nervous system first implying that information flows in the direction of gravity from the brain down to the rest of the body.

However, if back in the late 1970s/early 1980s, when those of us in the field were discussing what do we call this, it's more than just physiology, had we'd known then what we know now, I am quite sure that perhaps a name immuno-neurology, immuno-psychology would have been given equal consideration, because what we are dealing with is a bi-directional highway. An even better would not imply that one part of a system is more important than the other. That would be the best solution.

There is no question that the original words psychoneuroimmunology denoting the nervous system is appropriate. Certainly emotions can have a profound impact upon the functioning of the immune system. There's absolutely no question about it that when you go through a divorce, when you are facing the prospect of losing your job, you lose a loved one, that is when you are more likely to come down with an infection and we know that happens. It's been documented in numerous studies.

Dr. Ron Glaser and Jan Kiecolt-Glaser at Ohio State University did some of the most convincing experiments starting with medical students who they found were more likely to have reactivation of herpes at the time of a major exam. Herpes is a ubiquitous virus in the American population; 90% of people have it. You might not have had an outbreak of a fever blister on your face since you were in grade school, but if you have ever had it, you've still got the virus.

That virus is hanging out in the ganglion of your trigeminal nerve and as long as your immune system is robust, it stays there. But when the immune system becomes compromised as it might when a student is pulling an all-nighter preparing for an exam, that is when the virus is able to start trotting out along the axon eventually to appear at the same place each time, which is where the nerve projects onto the skin. And then once the immune system gets itself together, the virus goes back into remission awaiting the next opportunity.

The way that the Glasers measured this outcome was not waiting for a fever blister. That rarely happens. They measured antibody titers because when the innate immune system was no longer able to keep the virus in check, it was allowed to start marching. It started marching along the nerves resulting in activation of the adaptive immune system. The cell stimulation resulted in the production of antibodies, so by measuring the antibodies, it told them that the immune system was compromised. The innate immune system was not able to keep them in that preclinical phase and the A team, as I referred to it earlier, the T-cells and the B-cells, were now mobilized.

They did another study with Alzheimer caregivers. For a spousal caregiver especially, this may very well be a 24/7 job and chances are that caregiver is elderly as well. The Glasers found that when these folks were vaccinated against influenza the antibody titer wasn't really that impressive, barely enough to be protective. That's no surprise. We've been teaching medical students for decades don't waste your time vaccinating someone when they're going through a divorce or some other emotional upheaval in their lives. Wait until they get on an even keel. You want to make sure the immune system is robust enough that you can get plenty of memory cells and antibodies being formed. No, that really wasn't a surprise.

What was a surprise is that five years after the loved one had gone into a nursing home or had passed away, the person was still immuno-compromised, reaffirming the definition of aging, which is the inability to rapidly recover from stress. That applies to the immune system as well. What might have been a hassle in our 20s and 30s becomes a really big deal in our 70s and 80s. Part of the reason is that it takes longer for the part of the brain that regulates cortisol to get it under control; and that part of the brain happens to be the hippocampus, the same part of the brain that consolidates information into memory.

So it's not surprising that as we get older not only do we become forgetful, but at the same time we suffer more illnesses related to stress. That includes increased incidence of pneumonia and other upper opportunistic infections due to an immune system that is not able to recover as quickly from setbacks people experience.

Many people have multiple sclerosis and it's not uncommon that during times of emotional upheaval that that individual is likely to have a flare-up of symptoms. Now how can that be? How can it be that emotional upheaval can down-regulate the immune system, leaving you vulnerable to infection, but at the same time cause a flare-up of an illness due to too much immunity? Wouldn't you predict that if stress makes one condition worse, it really ought to make the other better? There is no contradiction. There is a very simple explanation, but before I explain that, there is one more thing you need to understand. Invariably the flare-up of the symptoms associated with multiple sclerosis occurs after the stress has happened, not before, not during, but afterwards.

Let's talk about what's happening here. The immune system covers a huge range. If you examine the normal white count values there is not a single number, there is a range within which the immune system can fall and the person can be perfectly healthy. That applies to a lot of things, but especially the immune system. It doesn't matter what is being examined, the level of ocytocine or mitogenesis or anything else.

Let's imagine for just a moment that everyone is normal, everyone in a room is normal at least in regards to the immune system; and let's imagine that the normal immune system ranges from the ceiling down to the floor. If the immune system goes down below the floor, that's the threshold below which it can't protect you. If your immune system goes up above the ceiling, that's the threshold above which you are likely to have a flare-up of multiple sclerosis or any other autoimmune disease.

Given the fact that everyone in the room is normal means that everyone is going to be within those bounds; the majority will be in the mid-range. But because of the immune response gene some people may have an immune system still in the normal range, but down close to the floor. Others will be up by the ceiling. Let's first consider what happens during stress.

First, for the people whose immune system is down close to the floor, Ron Glaser's medical students, for example, the pressure is building. Fear of failure sets in. They start burning the midnight oil. They don't take time to sleep properly. They don't prepare healthy foods. They don't have time to exercise and as I explained earlier, their immune systems are on the rocks.

Therefore cortisol is going up and as result of the anxiety epinephrine is going up. As they worry about blowing this exam it pushes their immune system down below that threshold. That is when they get sick. During this time of stress is when the immune system fails and the person comes down with an infection.

Now the exam is over. Not only did the student pass, they did quite well. Cortisol comes down, allowing the immune system to come back up, except at this point something very interesting happens. The same thing that happened the last time you ate a candy bar in the mid-afternoon in order to get a little energy to make it through the rest of the day. Many people have done that and have discovered that 30 minutes to an hour afterwards they have no energy. They almost go into a coma. They crash. Here's why.

It's after lunch. The pancreas finished its job of putting the sugar from lunch into storage long ago. It's taking a nap. It doesn't have to work again until dinnertime. It opens up its eye to see what time it is and sees this wall of sugar coming at it. It panics, where did this come from? It starts cranking up large amounts of insulin to put this sugar coming at it into storage. It doesn't want to get caught with its pants down again, so just in case there's another candy bar coming, the pancreas produces a little bit extra except there is no second candy bar. So what does the extra insulin do?

It puts the sugar you need to function into storage. Your blood sugar will actually drop down below where it was when you started dropping those coins into the vending machine. So what do you do? You eat another candy bar and start the whole cycle all over again. This is the rule in biology. It's called overcompensation.

When a system is out of adjustment for a long time or if it changes very abruptly as it attempts to come back to homeostasis, it overcompensates. We see it not only with the insulin response after putting a huge amount of refined sugar into the system, we see it with the action potential at the nerve ending, hypo and hyperpolarization. We see it with the cortisol response after the cortisol is being elevated for an extended time as it comes back down to more its normal, it drops down below normal before coming back up. And when it drops down below normal, that's when it's going to allow the immune system to bounce up higher than it normally would be.

That's not a bad thing. It allows it to mop up whatever residual virus may still be hanging around, but let's consider the person who is genetically vulnerable to autoimmune disease whose immune system is up at the ceiling. During the stress that same elevated level of cortisol pushes their immune system down into the mid-range; and yes a lot of people with these types of illnesses do report that during times of stress their autoimmune systems are more easily managed. But when the stress is over, the cortisol comes down. It overcompensates in layering the immune system, which is normally up there to go above the ceiling and that's why the flare-up of the symptoms will always occur after the stress is over.

We're dealing with a normal rise and fall in cortisol and a corresponding fall and rise in the immune system. Depending upon the microenvironment in which it occurs, whether the immune system started high or started low, it's going to dictate what kind of clinical outcome is likely to occur. The question you are probably asking is what can I do about it if my immune is up there close to the ceiling leaving me vulnerable to autoimmune or inflammatory disease, how can I bring it down? Or if my immune system is down there by the floor, how can

I bring up into the healthy mid-range? That's the wrong question to be asking.

I told you that I would be sacrificing some accuracy for the sake of clarity and I've been doing that here. Let's fix it. To be accurate about things, there is no single immune system. Think in terms of plural, the immune systems. Remember what I told you about the specificity of the immune system when your T-cells when your B-cells are engaged in a form of friendly fire when you're cranking out antibodies directed against the myelin sheath, it is only those cells that are specific for the myelin protein that are overactive not the others. And they may comprise only 2% of your total lymphocytes, so it's only 2% of your cells that are actually up there at the ceiling. The rest of your immune system may be down in the healthy mid-range, the ones that you need to fight off influenza or rhinovirus; and you may have some cells that are down close to the floor, perhaps the ones that are normally designed to take on Gram-negative bacteria for example.

Realize, too, that because the 2% of your cells are working 24/7, 365 days a year trying to get rid of something that will never go away because it's part of you, they may be using up more than their fair share of a finite resource. You may have functional immune-efficiency even though you have a normal complement of cells. The question to ask is what can I do to bring this little piece of my immune system down, that 2% of my cells, but only that part? Leave the rest of it alone and by the way, don't bring it down too far, while at the same time bring this little piece of my immune system down by the floor up, but again not too far and at exactly the same time leave all of the other cells where they're supposed to be alone.

And the answer to that question is nothing. There's nothing in the pharmacy. There's nothing in the health food store that works with that degree of precision.

We know an awful lot about the immune system and how it works, but nowhere near the amount of information that we will need to have to go in and manipulate it with a degree of precision required to bring about the desired outcome. The drugs that are currently used to treat arthritis and bursitis, such as prednisone, dexamethasone, and hydrocortisone work in a shot gun manner. They'll bring the whole immune system down, which is why when you take those drugs, you've got to be very careful to avoid exposure to pathogens and for quite a long time afterwards. There are some drugs like cyclosporin A, which are used by transplant surgeons, that are a little more specific in that they tend to down-regulate T-helper cells., However, they don't distinguish between the T-helper cell that is likely to reject the transplant and the T-helper cell that is needed to help fight off influenza.

There is a huge amount of research going on. Scientists are trying to develop designer antibodies to target very specific receptors. They are trying to come up with modified forms of cytokines, trying to manipulate their receptors, so they get rid of the harmful effects yet preserve the beneficial ones. There is a lot at stake, including a Nobel Prize.

It will be an extremely important discovery. Once we learn to manipulate the immune system with that degree of precision, the chapter in medical books called Transplantation Immunology, the chapter called Infectious Disease, the chapter on Inflammation, and the one dealing with Autoimmunity, will all be reduced to a single paragraph which you will now find in the chapter called The History of Medicine, but right now we don't have that option.

I told you that there is nothing that can be done to modulate the immune system with that degree of precision. Now I'm going to take that back. I hate to endorse anything, especially things that have to do with nutrition, because there is so much misinformation out there. There is a lot of preliminary information and the experiments ongoing, so we just don't know yet the validity of many of the claims being made, especially about various supplements. However, there is something available that you can do based upon nutrition which seems to work in exactly the way that you would desire to. It will bring down the path of the immune system that needs to be brought down, bring up the part that needs to be brought up, and leave the rest of it alone.

That solution is to reduce caloric intake. Now this is not a new discovery. It is often presented in the media as being a new revelation. The fact is the research has dated back to the 1960s when Dr. Roy Walford was conducting research at what later became the National Institutes on Aging. However he was working with mice and rats. He was working with laboratory models and a lot of people can't relate to rodents, so much of that research was largely ignored.

What he found though was that by reducing caloric intake, the animals lived longer and in the intervening decades the studies have been replicated in a number of species. Perhaps the most renowned immunologist of the past generation is Dr. Robert Good whose name was synonymous with the entire field of transplantation immunology when he was at the National Institutes of Health. He dedicated the last ten years of his research career trying to find out why it is that when you restrict the caloric intake of both humans and animals it appears to restore harmony to their immune system. If a person or animal is susceptible to diseases associated with too much immunity or too little, caloric restriction makes the symptoms more manageable.

There are other benefits as well. There's a lot of research to suggest that there are changes occurring within the body consistent with caloric reduction that might prolong life. The question is exactly what is mediating this increased life expectancy and what are some of the data that would indicate that reducing caloric intake might in humans prolong life expectancy? It would be very difficult to conduct the lifetime studies in human beings.

You couldn't ethically do this study, due to the risk of malnutrition. After being asked to restrict their dietary intake over a period of years, even decades, probably a lot of people would not comply.

However, there has been enough interest that some preliminary studies have been conducted and it has been found that reducing caloric intake results in a decrease in fat storage and mass. It also results in a decrease in blood glucose levels and the establishment of a healthy ratio of the lipids low density lipo-protein (LDL) to high density lipo-protein (HDL). You want more of the HDL, which tends to transport the cholesterol from the cells back to the liver and less of the so called bad cholesterol, the LDL. Caloric restriction decreases the LDLs, the bad cholesterol and increases the HDLs. It also results in a decrease in core body temperature, which is a reflection of overall decreased metabolism and it can result in a decrease in blood pressure.

Decreased energy expenditure beyond that expected for the amount of weight that has been lost suggests that there is some general reduction in overall metabolic rate. People who restrict their caloric intake have also been found to have less oxidated stress. Earlier I discussed free radicals and how these unstable molecules tend to steal electrons from healthy tissues. There is a reduction in that phenomenon in people who reduce their caloric intake. There is a reduction in the amount of damage done to DNA, something which can occur during the course of our lives. There is also less chronic inflammation in people who reduce their calories and there are changes in various hormone levels that appear to be protective.

So how would this work? Several explanations have been offered. One is that by reducing the metabolism of food there is a reduction in the overall production of free radicals. Remember free radicals are also known as oxidated metabolites, so if there's less metabolism being driven by oxygen, then a person will have fewer of these free radicals being produced. And as I noted earlier free radicals have been associated with a large number of illnesses including things like cancer and heart disease, which can kill people and shorten life span.

A second explanation which is not mutually exclusive from the one I just mentioned is that when you eat less, you are more motivated to exercise. Basically you are foraging for food. If you visit the zoo just before feeding time, that's when you'll find the animals scurrying all over the place. The monkeys are leaping from one end of the enclosure to another. The big cat is pacing back and forth. We know that there are extraordinary benefits of exercise, some of which we covered just in the context of the immune system.

But this information is useless. What exactly is less? How do you interpret this guidance, reduce your calorie intake? Reduce it compared with what benchmark? Less is a relative term, so less of what?

Maybe you are already eating exactly what you need to be eating. For you to eat less would put you into the malnourished zone. Or perhaps you don't eat enough and so you might be a person who needs to eat more to reach that point of less and wouldn't that be great? So exactly what constitutes less?

Try this experiment. Take a baby rat, separate him from the litter just about the time that he would normally be weaned. Put him in a back room and then buy a 50 pound bag of Purina "Rat Chow." Fill a bowl full of food and allow that rat to eat whenever he wants. Now each day weigh how much food remains. You want to calculate exactly the number of grams that that rat eats during a 24-hour period and make sure the food is always there. When he wakes up from a deep sleep, the food is there for him to eat. He can eat whenever wants during the day or his equivalent of night.

Now let's say for the sake of illustration that your rat eats ten grams everyday. That is what a nutritionist would call his free feeding diet. It is the amount of food that a person or an animal will eat with no restriction. Now cut back the food, give him seven or eight grams. Give him a diet that is comprised of 20% or even 30% fewer calories than he would eat given a choice. Within one week your rat will develop a nice shiny coat. He'll develop resistance to Sendai virus, which is the rat equivalent of herpes, ubiquitous among wild rats, and he'll go on to live significantly longer than your neighbor's rat who gets to eat whenever he wants.

Human beings that live in opulent societies like certain parts of America and the animals those people keep as pets are probably the only creatures on this planet that get to enjoy a free-feeding dict. It's very unnatural. Most cultures and certainly wild animals do not have this luxury, although I'm not sure it really should be considered a luxury given the fact that it's probably going to hasten the person's demise if they eat incessantly.

There are two ways that you can reduce your caloric intake. You can consult nutrition textbooks and chances are because a lot of the guidelines are written on the basis of what the average person does the recommendations that you will find are predicated upon a person eating a free feeding diet. A lot of people believe that some of the recommendations about our nutritional needs are actually inflated. It is more than we really need if we want to achieve a state of optimal health. Of course if your nutrition textbook has already taken into account what I'm speaking about, if it is discussed in the introductory chapters, then of course follow the guidelines.

However, most texts do not consider this so when you peruse the table that tells you how many calories you need on a given day based upon your age, gender, lifestyle, take that number, but only consume 20% of it because chances are that is where you would need to be in order to achieve that state of optimal health. That is one way of doing it.

You can go to a nice restaurant with your little calorie counter, which tells you how many calories are associated with each of the ingredients on that plate, then ask to speak with the chef to find out exactly what ingredients were used to prepare the meal. Make yourself absolutely obnoxious. Or you can do it in a much better way and that is separate your needs from your wants. When you want seconds, you want thirds, but you don't really need it, push the plate away. When there's a slight edge on your appetite, you really want more, but you don't have to have it, that is probably going to put you right where you need to be.

And the best part about this is it takes into account daily variability. Obviously if you spend half the morning shoveling your car out of a snow bank or mowing the lawn before going off to work, then you will have spent many more calories staying warm and expending on yourself that day compared with a day when you might be lying on the couch watching a national championship sporting event. Use that rule and you will find yourself exactly where you need to be.

The reduction in caloric intake is probably going to address your hunger, after all you are going to be eating what you need. However, it is what you *want* that's going to be impacted. After a period of time it might be difficult to consistently comply with this regimen and recognizing this, some have come up with alternative ways of doing this, which seem to have very similar benefits.

One is the practice of intimate fasting. Sometimes it's referred to as every-other-day feeding or alternate-day fasting. This approach does not reduce the overall average number of calories that a person takes in. It simply alters the pattern of food intake. This has been found in animals to prolong life span and also to improve a large number of metabolic measures of health. It hasn't been as well studied as caloric restriction. However intimate and fasting has been found to result in beneficial changes in insulin levels as well as glucose status. In some studies it has been found to be correlated with improved blood lipid levels, as well as a reduction in blood pressure in humans.

Another interpretation is that caloric restriction may reduce the total amount of protein coming into the diet. The average American eats considerably more protein than is really recommended. In fact Americans eat 15% to 17% of their total daily calories in the form of protein. Studies have shown that when protein is restricted to no more than 10% of energy intake, this can result in a decrease in the onset of cancer along with other health benefits. It may be that one need not reduce total calories, but just a matter of reducing the total amount of protein.

There is also evidence that exercise will induce leanness that may slow the aging process as well without the need for caloric restriction. So again as I mentioned before, it may not be just the energy reduction that extends the life span, but the overall energy balance that a person maintains whereby now the exercise is burning off the additional calories.

There is one more intriguing interpretation which is that the cells in your body learn to handle stress when you are reducing caloric intake. Obviously if there's a slight edge on your appetite the cells are going to be exposed to a form of stress: adversity. This would fall into the category of use stress, or good stress. One of the arguments is that when the cells are accustomed to that need for a little more, when a big stress comes along, they can basically shrug it off and say been there, done that, got the t-shirt, no problem.

In the context of stress management I refer to this as cross-stressing when a person learns to recover from stress in one context, it becomes easier to deal with it and recover quickly in other contexts. And so some scientists have now taken this concept and applied it at the cellular level. As I mentioned before, none of these interpretations is mutually exclusive. The bottom line is it doesn't really matter what the mechanism is whereby it's working. The studies clearly show that when a person reduces their intake of calories there is an improvement in their metabolic health and in the animal studies an improvement and increase in life expectancy.

Summary Recommendations

've provided you with a lot of information in this book, some of it you can start using and applying in your life. Other information simply explains how systems work; and I went into some detail explaining that because I firmly believe that when you understand what's going on behind the biological scenes, it makes it much easier to comply and actually follow through and do what is rec ommended. You become an informed consumer enabled to make better choices and evaluate those things that really might be beneficial and those that are simply fads, which may have limited benefit if any at all.

I would now like to basically summarize the key points that will enable you to achieve a state of optimal health and ways to stay well. First of all I will note that the Centers for Disease Control have noted that chronic disease is responsible for seven of every ten deaths in

America; chronic disease is responsible for 70% of the deaths. But more relevant is the fact that there are just four behaviors that you have total control over that are responsible for that chronic disease. They are lack of physical activity, poor nutrition, tobacco use, and excessive consumption of alcohol.

If you want to live to a ripe-old age, if you want to have maximum functional capacity right up until the day you die, then these are the things that you need be doing. Engage in a minimum of 30 minutes of moderate exercise every day of the week. Earlier I said three days a week is okay, as do many of the guidelines. That is the minimum. The reason we say three days a week or three to five days a week is that a person is more likely to be compliant if they only have to do something three to five days a week. So in order to increase the likelihood of compliance, a more realistic guideline is offered in the hope that people are more likely to do it.

However if you are able to exercise seven days a week a minimum of 30 minutes, each of those days is essential. This doesn't mean that you have to sign away your first born child or take out a second mortgage on your home in order to afford a membership in local gym. No, exercise is the form of walking briskly from your car into a building. It's using the stairs instead of the elevator. It's the movement we engage in doing everyday activities. That is exercise.

Consume a diet based upon the dietary guidelines for Americans, the My Plate protocol, which is now replacing the pyramid scheme. Basically the recommendations are those that comprise the Mediterranean or Asian diet. This is a plant based diet with a reduction in overall protein, meat served on a monthly basis, lean meat, and fish on a weekly basis. Most of the plate is covered in multi-colored legumes, leafy vegetables, fruits and whole grain bread.

Maintain a healthful weight. If you smoke or for that matter if you use any tobacco product, then stop. If you don't smoke, then don't start. If you consumer alcohol, do so in moderation and that means no more than two drinks on a daily basis for men and no more than one drink per day for women. The reason is because men have more alcohol dehydrogenases than women do. They have a great capacity to metabolize the alcohol and so that is why the recommendation is different.

If you do these very simple things you will benefit not only your immune system, but your heart, your brain, your endocrine system, every aspect of your physiology. And you will indeed achieve the state of optimal health that you so richly deserve.

Note from the Author

Thank you for reading *How To Feel Better*. In this book, we have been exploring immunity and the relationship with the brain chemicals and your thoughts and feelings. You may be asking, who is Nick Hall? And why is he qualified to teach me about such an important topic as this? Let me give you a bit of my background as it relates to this topic.

After spending two years researching stress-related communication patterns in whales and dolphins for the Office of Naval Research, I went to graduate school where I completed studies in Neuroscience and then post-doctoral training in Immunology. I then spent the better part of 30 years researching the chemical pathways linking the brain with the immune system. The field is called Psychoneuroimmunology and over the years my NIH funded research ran the gambit from assessing the use of guided imagery in cancer patients, to how malnutrition and exercise impact the brain and immune system. I now spend most of my time applying this research with elite athletes and corporate clients at the Saddlebrook Resort Wellness Center, which I direct. I also teach Human Nutrition at the University of South Florida College Of Nursing.

And now, after reading this book, I hope you find it will be time to take action.

Printed in the USA
CPSIA information can be obtained
at www.ICGtesting.com
JSHW012036140824
68134JS00033B/3083

9 781722 500160